GW00649722

Copyright © 2022 Rob Verkerk, Meleni Aldridge and Melissa Smith

The moral right of the author has been asserted.

Apart from any fair dealing for the purposes of research or private study, or criticism or review, as permitted under the Copyright, Designs and Patents Act 1988, this publication may only be reproduced, stored or transmitted, in any form or by any means, with the prior permission in writing of the publishers, or in the case of reprographic reproduction in accordance with the terms of licences issued by the Copyright Licensing Agency. Enquiries concerning reproduction outside those terms should be sent to the publishers.

Matador
Unit E2 Airfield Business Park,
Harrison Road, Market Harborough,
Leicestershire. LE16 7UL
Tel: 0116 2792299
Email: books@troubador.co.uk
Web: www.troubador.co.uk/matador
Twitter: @matadorbooks

ISBN 978 1803130 194

British Library Cataloguing in Publication Data.
A catalogue record for this book is available from the British Library.

Printed and bound by CPI Group (UK) Ltd, Croydon, CR0 4YY

Matador is an imprint of Troubador Publishing Ltd

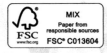

DEDICATION

This book is dedicated to the many health seekers who have continued to set out on new health paths, filled with hope and positivity, only to find themselves at yet another dead end.

Health creation is multifaceted and multidimensional. The pivot point for our physical health, the foundation of vital resilience, always has been and for some time hence, will remain — the way we interact with the food we eat. Our connection to food is one of the most important relationships we have in life. Like any relationship that is valued, nurtured and respected, it holds the potential to dramatically change our lives for the better.

Editor

Meleni Aldridge BSc NutrMed Dip cPNI Cert LTFHE

Contributors

Robert Verkerk BSc MSc DIC PhD FACN
Meleni Aldridge BSc NutrMed Dip cPNI Cert LTHFE
Melissa Smith Dip ION
Mike Abbott
Copyrighted material

Cover design by Tacon Design Ltd

Design and artwork by Charlie Jones

Alliance for Natural Health International
Old Station House
78 Dorking Road
Chilworth
Surrey
GU4 8NS
United Kingdom

www.anhinternational.org
All enquiries to: info@anhinternational.org

DISCLAIMER

The information contained within this eBook is for educational purposes only and does not constitute medical advice. If you have any underlying health issues or concerns, we strongly advise that you consult with a suitably qualified and experienced health professional before making any changes to your diet or lifestyle.

Reset Eating: Turn Your Food Into Powerful Medicine To Reset Your Health & Resilience.

ENDORSEMENTS

The current pandemic is a call-to-action for a self-care reset. Rob Verkerk PhD and Meleni Aldridge from the Alliance for Natural Health International deliver a timely, thoroughly science-based review of the practical strategies we can employ to reclaim our resilience.

Ronald Hoffman, MD, CNS
Host of the Intelligent Medicine podcast (www.drhoffman.com)

Food in our day-to-day life is often not given much thought, it's something we reach for when hungry. But there is great power in food. The old view is that food supplies energy and 39 essential nutrients. The new view is that food is a source of over 10,000 substances that profoundly influence health within hours of a single meal. Food and nutritional medicine have the power to transform your health and are safe, affordable, and accessible. Food satiates us, but also connects us, inspires us, and quite literally transforms us. This guide will empower and inspire you.

Benjamin I. Brown, ND
Director, The Nutritional Medicine Institute, UK

Contributing Editor, Integrative Health and Applied Nutrition

Advisory Board and Lecturer, BCNH College of Nutrition and Health

Today our food policies and governmental nutrition recommendations are influenced by agricultural conglomerates and their lobbyists. It is no mistake that highly processed junk food and overconsumption of sugar are not censored by these supposed experts resulting in out-of-control chronic disease. Yet clear and relevant nutrition guidelines are at our fingertips provided by the Alliance for Natural Health International. The Reset Eating eBook from ANH International provides scientifically rigorous recommendations, guidelines for food choices, and tools for meal preparation all within interactive links. Healthful living through sound choices of good food, the foundation of life, is yours by choosing Reset Eating!

Jeanne A Drisko, MD, CNS, FACN
Professor Emeritus, University of Kansas Medical Center, USA

ACKNOWLEDGEMENTS

This book contains decades of combined independent learning from Rob and I (Mel); Rob as a scientist, myself as a nutritional practitioner and clinical psychoneuroimmunologist, both of us as victims of inappropriate diets and misdirected conventional treatments at earlier ages. On top of that, there's the nearly two decades of development, training and education that we've been leading while heading the non-profit, the Alliance for Natural Health (ANH) International. For that part, we're incredibly grateful to Melissa for all the support and wisdom she's offered over her years with ANH — and her immense passion, also sparked from her own health challenges and journey to wellness. We're also incredibly grateful to the many contributions by Michelle Hallworth over the last decade in finding better ways of communicating complex information about human diets and behaviour from an evolutionary perspective — in a language that anyone can understand.

Public health has not only inadequately identified the dietary patterns, behaviours and addictions that cause the majority of preventable chronic diseases, it has also failed to empower health creation among individuals and communities. It's clear that the majority of public health messaging is influenced more by corporate pressure than reasoned medical, clinical or scientific evidence. It also tends to be prescriptive and one-size-fits-all, being poorly adapted to the needs, environments, cultures and genes of the individual in question. This book provides a new way of looking at the interaction between our food, our genes and our bodies, recognising that food is so much more than a source of energy. If it's any one thing, it's a source of information for the body that drives genetic expression to create health rather than nurture disease.

Whilst food is not by any means the only contributor to health, its role — as a reflection of the most intimate way in which the insides of our bodies interact with the outside world — provides a fundamental cornerstone to health, one that has unfortunately been relegated to the margins of mainstream medicine.

Humans, being multi-dimensional by nature, require multifactorial solutions to restore balance when it has been lost. In creating total health and resilience, nutrition must of course be partnered by many other things. Among them are mission, purpose, community, physical activity, stress transformation, sleep quality and spiritual connection.

This work would not be here in this format without the skill and creativity of Charlie Jones whose design and artwork has brought our words to life when words were just not enough. Mike Abbott and Ismail Faryad, from our media unit, helped deliver some great graphics and Gemma Tacon did her magic on the cover design. We must again mention Michelle Hallworth's input, in this case, her final editorial input — we don't call her the 'grammar police' for nothing. John Vincent's inspiration and energy continue to guide us on many fronts and — thank you, John — for providing such a poignant Foreword.

Next, we must thank all the ANH supporters around the world over the years for their contributions. Without the feedback and incredible stories from those who've transformed their health

by following our guidance, this book would never have made it to publication. That includes the many nutritional and practitioner associations and individual practitioners who've followed our work, provided us feedback — and all those who've been following our journey through Food4Health and keto-adaptation over the last decade.

A heartfelt thank you to all of you for being on the journey with us.

Finally, we need to thank from the bottom of our hearts, our families and friends for being so loving, accepting and supportive of our mission. Words are never enough.

Meleni Aldridge
BSc NutrMed Dip cPNI Cert LTHFE

Robert Verkerk
BSc MSc DIC PhD FACN

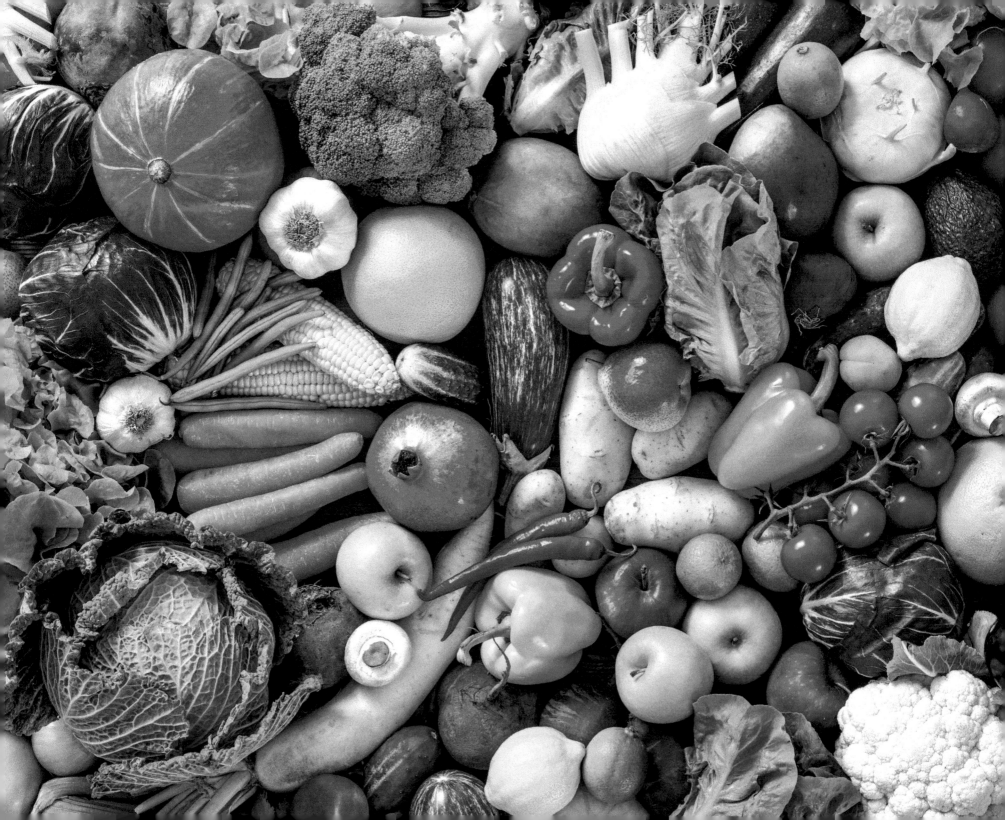

EATING THE F4H WAY: A FEW KICKSTARTER RECIPES

V VEGAN / CAN BE MADE VEGAN

INTRODUCTION

Eating a healthy and balanced diet is key to improving the quality of your life, especially when coupled with regular physical activity and due attention to your emotional health. Right?

It seems so simple, yet government guidelines and public health messages are still falling so far short of the mark when it comes to properly supporting health and wellness. We like to talk in terms of health creation, rather than disease management. And food is the foundation to it all because food is not merely fuel or an energy carrier, it's information too.

We felt so strongly about the fact that government guidelines and public health campaigns were simply not delivering, we were compelled to produce our own guideline 'plate' that represents food group composition over a typical day. It's a 'plate' that's rooted in extensive nutritional science, clinical and citizen experience, but more than that, it's anti-inflammatory, keto-adapted and will help you develop - or maintain - metabolic (and immunological) flexibility. Metabolic flexibility,

which in simple terms is your ability to switch efficiently between fat and carbs as your primary energy carriers, creates resilience, crucial for resisting disease and creating health. Our ancestral norm if you will. A state of being we like to call 'flexi-keto'.

We've called it the Food4Health 'plate', because that's what it does. But in trying to come up with a short, punchy descriptor to give a bit more detail, we've failed miserably. So, this is what we're left with — a largely unprocessed, relatively low carb/high complex carb, low glycaemic, moderately high fat and protein-rich, anti-inflammatory, pro-mitochondrial, longevity plate that sets the scene for metabolic, and also, immune system flexibility!

What follows is a starting point and a rough guideline to help you on your journey to being a keto-adapted, super-resilient, metabolically flexible and immunologically well person. Our bodies have a rather miraculous capacity for self-healing when we feed them with the right 'information'.

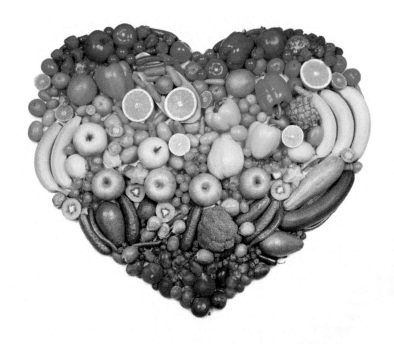

We hope your food journey is inspiring, enlightening and rekindles, or strengthens, your most important relationship. The one with your own body.

Enjoy!

©2022 ALLIANCE FOR NATURAL HEALTH INTERNATIONAL

FOREWORD

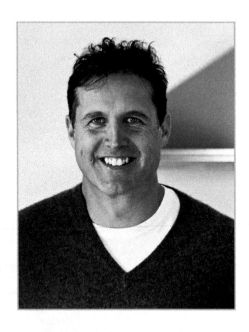

John Vincent MBE
*Co-Founder of LEON Restaurants,
Co-author of School Food Plan
(UK) & Entrepreneur*

I am as excited that this book has been written as I hope you will be.

It has been created by the Alliance for Natural Health (ANH-Intl), people who I have got to know well in my time running LEON and working on projects like the School Food Plan. The team who lead ANH are scientists and nutritionists determined to help us all learn from the available science and from the clinical experience of the world's leading medical practitioners.

They have written this book to provide an impartial and in-depth guide for what to actually do. And explain why and how they have come to this conclusion.

You will find the latest insights into why food works in different ways in different bodies, why some people can thrive on veggie food and others can't, why some people have difficulty burning fat, and others don't, and why snacking can be deadly.

And it recognises that we've still got genes that are very similar to those of our palaeolithic ancestors, yet we live in a world with convenience stores, processed foods, and refined carbs on every street corner.

The book gets under the covers of what's driving the silent pandemic of metabolic diseases like diabetes and obesity. And why people suffering from these diseases have been the most vulnerable to Covid-19.

Many doctors and nutritionists look to ANH for guidance and for the most up to date science. So, it is a great milestone that they have produced a book of their own.

Rob, Mel and Melissa don't just say 'do as we say' – I know from my own longstanding relationship with them that they are role-models for the actions and behaviours set out in these pages. So, you won't be asked to follow a practically impossible theory.

This is the book I have been waiting for, for a long time.

I wish you well in making a habit of putting these lessons and insights into practice.

You will feel better and be better to feel...

©2022 ALLIANCE FOR NATURAL HEALTH INTERNATIONAL

Laying the table...

Different people's lifestyles and genetic make-up call for flexibility in any system of guidelines. One size, unfortunately, does not fit all. So, guidelines should be seen as something of a starting point or a rough guide, not a 'bible'. Fine-tuning over time is generally needed and you may also find the process enhanced by working with a nutrition health professional.

However, as a first step — getting your food composition into balance with your evolutionary heritage, avoiding damaged and ultra-processed foods, removing foods to which you're sensitive, and reducing your dependence on refined carbs, can deliver results that can be felt in a matter of days.

In taking this first step, we have to understand important areas of current government guidelines that don't reflect the most up-to-date nutritional science. We have outlined our top 10 concerns with government guidelines below:

1. Starchy carbs are massively over-recommended

2. The effect on glycaemic load of food processing technologies and cooking is generally ignored (how consumed carbs affect your blood sugar level)

3. Low-fat is still advocated, despite it often being linked to diets high in refined carbs and sugars

4. Grains (eg, cereals, bread, pasta) are recommended as the primary source of energy, despite numerous problems, especially with wheat and gluten, ranging from coeliac disease, leaky gut syndrome, non-coeliac gluten-sensitivity and numerous other related gastro-intestinal and autoimmune conditions

5. Helping individuals out of food addiction, especially the combined effect of sugar and particular fats, is not adequately taken into account

6. There is inadequate emphasis placed on certain food groups, such as healthy fats and concentrated nutrients such as in herbs and spices

7. There is little or no consideration of meal/food frequency

8. There is little or no consideration of processing, preparation or cooking methods and how these can impact nutritional quality or add to your toxic burden

9. There is no provision for supplements, despite evidence of their value in many sub-populations (eg, Omega-3 fatty acids, vitamin D, multivitamin/minerals, etc)

10. Governments push dairy products to ensure sufficient calcium is consumed. Evidence shows that calcium is not normally deficient in the diet, but rather it is co-factors such as vitamin D, vitamin K2, magnesium and other nutrients that are in too short a supply. Humans did not evolve to consume large quantities of milk from other animals and lactase deficiency (lactose intolerance) is exceedingly common in some populations, ranging from 45-100% in Latin-American populations, to around 90% in many east Asian populations.

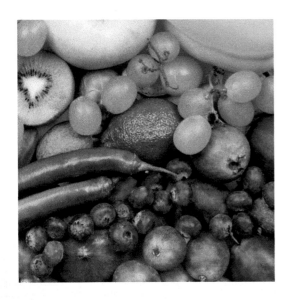

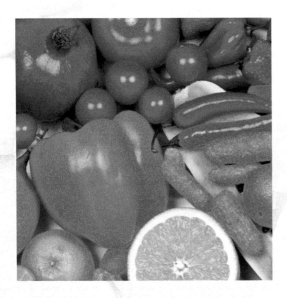

Critical to our health is the relative amounts and quality of macronutrients (proteins, fats and carbs), as well as micronutrients (vitamins, minerals, enzymes, phytonutrients etc), along with the state of these at the point they enter our bodies.

Alongside this, we have to consider meal frequency, and it is now widely recognised that the snacking culture, that has made it a norm to eat energy-dense foods between meals, not only contributes to excess calories, but also promotes low-grade inflammation that is at the basis of most chronic diseases. Fasting for 5 hours between meals is achievable for most people, albeit requiring a bit of self-discipline in the early stages of becoming a 'non-snacker'.

Moving from becoming an energy-dense consumer, to a nutrient-dense consumer, is definitely part of this journey. As is becoming less dependent on simple carbohydrates as your source of fuel. Throughout most of our ancestral past, we have utilised fats as a primary energy source, and rapidly expanding scientific research showing the weight loss, health and endurance benefits of a keto-adapted (higher fat/protein, low carb) diet can no longer be ignored.

Nutrition is of course just one of the pillars of health and wellness. Alongside the information on food in these pages, health creation also demands that you remember to be active regularly, manage your emotional health and prioritise adequate sleep.

Eat frugally, get physical, be mindful and rest properly is probably the best prescription for health that anyone could receive.

On this basis, and to help you with your dietary goals, our Food4Health guide represents the main food groups in your day's eating as a percentage by weight and shows this on a plate for visual reference.

For many people this is a more realistic representation that is more relevant to those interested in health creation than the system widely used by governments, which shows the food groups according to their energy (calorie) contribution.

©2022 ALLIANCE FOR NATURAL HEALTH INTERNATIONAL

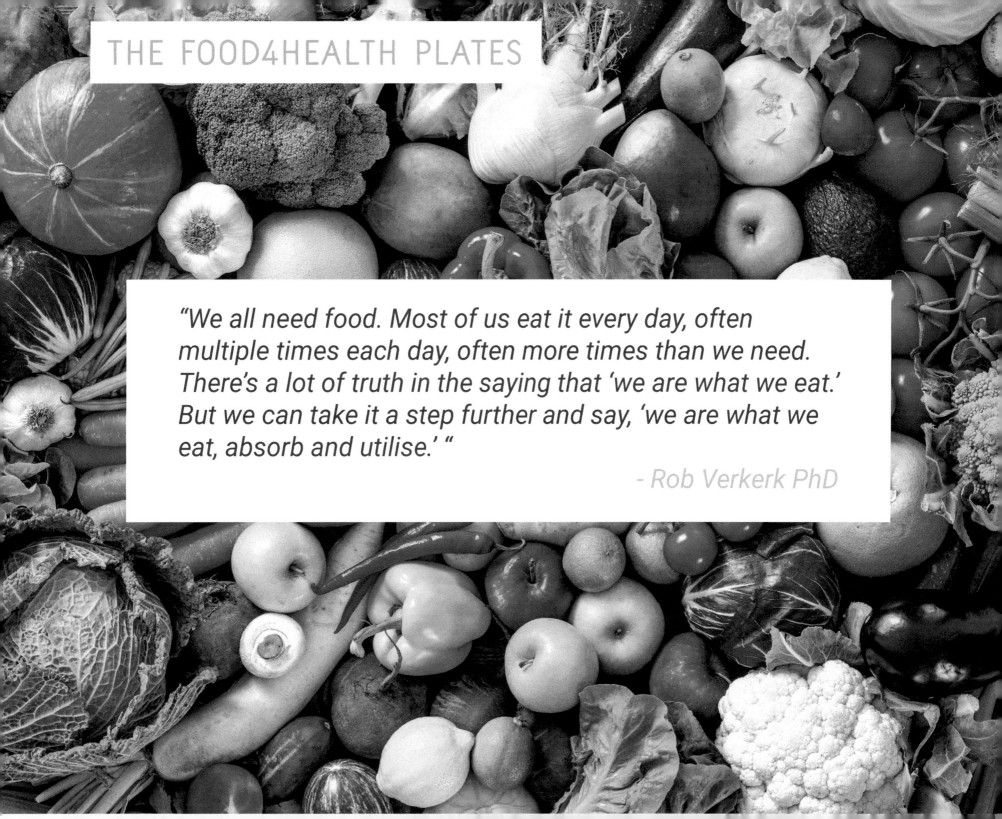

THE FOOD4HEALTH PLATES

"We all need food. Most of us eat it every day, often multiple times each day, often more times than we need. There's a lot of truth in the saying that 'we are what we eat.' But we can take it a step further and say, 'we are what we eat, absorb and utilise.' "

- Rob Verkerk PhD

Here are two of our food 'plates'. The first is our general flexitarian or omnivore 'plate' and on the following page is our Vegan 'plate', both representing a day's eating for adults.

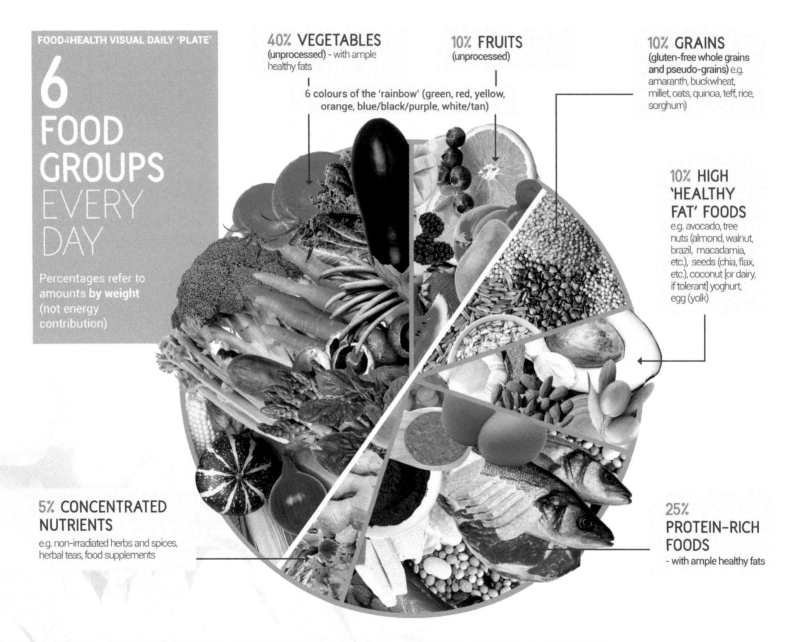

FOOD4HEALTH VISUAL DAILY 'PLATE'

6 FOOD GROUPS EVERY DAY

Percentages refer to amounts **by weight** (not energy contribution)

40% VEGETABLES
(unprocessed) - with ample healthy fats

6 colours of the 'rainbow' (green, red, yellow, orange, blue/black/purple, white/tan)

10% FRUITS
(unprocessed)

10% GRAINS
(gluten-free whole grains and pseudo-grains) e.g. amaranth, buckwheat, millet, oats, quinoa, teff, rice, sorghum)

10% HIGH 'HEALTHY FAT' FOODS
e.g. avocado, tree nuts (almond, walnut, brazil, macadamia, etc.), seeds (chia, flax, etc.), coconut [or dairy, if tolerant] yoghurt, egg (yolk)

25% PROTEIN-RICH FOODS
- with ample healthy fats

5% CONCENTRATED NUTRIENTS
e.g. non-irradiated herbs and spices, herbal teas, food supplements

FOOD4HEALTH GUIDE FOR FLEXITARIAN / OMNIVORE ADULTS
Please also refer to the associated 10 key guidelines on page 8.

 ©2022 ALLIANCE FOR NATURAL HEALTH INTERNATIONAL

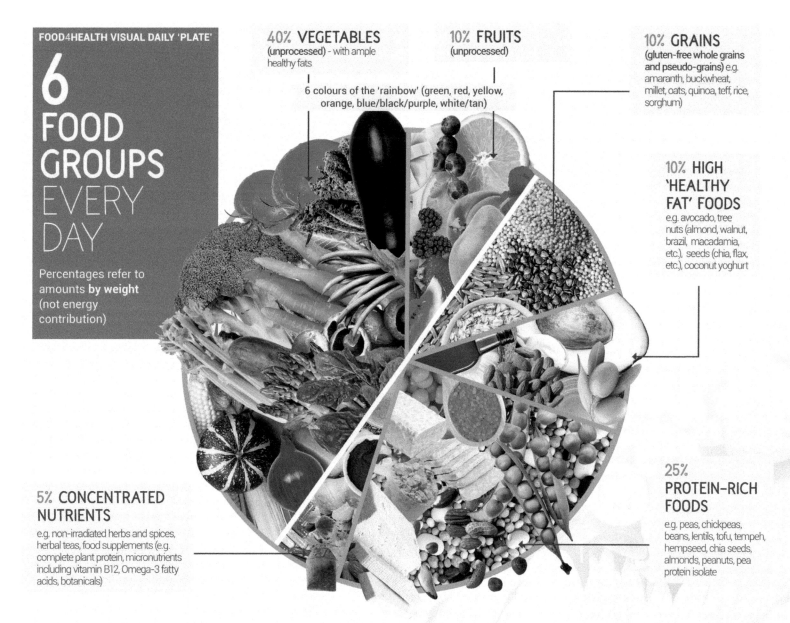

6 FOOD GROUPS EVERY DAY

Percentages refer to amounts **by weight** (not energy contribution)

40% VEGETABLES
(unprocessed) - with ample healthy fats

6 colours of the 'rainbow' (green, red, yellow, orange, blue/black/purple, white/tan)

10% FRUITS
(unprocessed)

10% GRAINS
(gluten-free whole grains and pseudo-grains) e.g. amaranth, buckwheat, millet, oats, quinoa, teff, rice, sorghum)

10% HIGH 'HEALTHY FAT' FOODS
e.g. avocado, tree nuts (almond, walnut, brazil, macadamia, etc.), seeds (chia, flax, etc.), coconut yoghurt

25% PROTEIN-RICH FOODS
e.g. peas, chickpeas, beans, lentils, tofu, tempeh, hempseed, chia seeds, almonds, peanuts, pea protein isolate

5% CONCENTRATED NUTRIENTS
e.g. non-irradiated herbs and spices, herbal teas, food supplements (e.g. complete plant protein, micronutrients including vitamin B12, Omega-3 fatty acids, botanicals)

FOOD4HEALTH GUIDE FOR VEGAN ADULTS

Please also refer to the associated 10 key guidelines on page 8.

Let's dig in

Both 'plates' are gluten and dairy free because these are the two most common allergens in the diet. You can add one or other back in if you know you can tolerate them. Gluten intolerance or sensitivity is often unnoticed for years, but can lead to all sorts of health problems from leaky gut to heart disease, cancer and diabetes.

This isn't what a single plate of your food will look like, it's your day's eating that's represented by weight, not by energy.

On the left of the big diagonal white line you've got all-important plant foods. And if you're looking at the flexitarian 'plate', you'll see some animal products too, and we advocate that these come from regenerative agriculture, not factory farming systems. Both 'plates' are still plant-based because so much of the food on them still comes from plants.

Plant foods & fruits

We include a large amount of veg and a relatively small amount of fruit. You should try to keep your veg and fruit in roughly a 4:1 ratio and don't lump them together. Fruits have a lot more sugar – albeit natural fructose, so need to be eaten in small quantities. The science tells us we shouldn't eat more sugar than 5% by energy of the total energy eaten in a day. Always try to eat your fruit whole and avoid fruit juices or too much dried fruit.

You should do your best to 'eat a rainbow every day' of all 6 different colours of Nature's phytonutrient groups, as recommended by the Institute for Functional Medicine. That means green, red, yellow, orange, blue/black/purple and white/tan/brown, which also creates a lot of diversity in your diet. Remember to mix it up with raw as well as lightly cooked vegetables. Veg can taste delicious with plenty of healthy fats, herbs and spices!

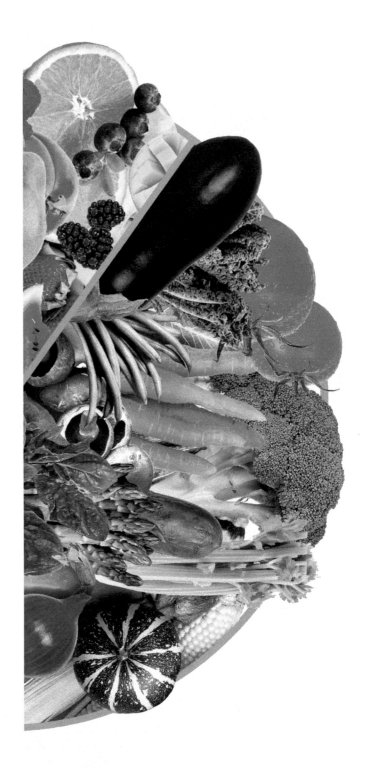

©2022 ALLIANCE FOR NATURAL HEALTH INTERNATIONAL

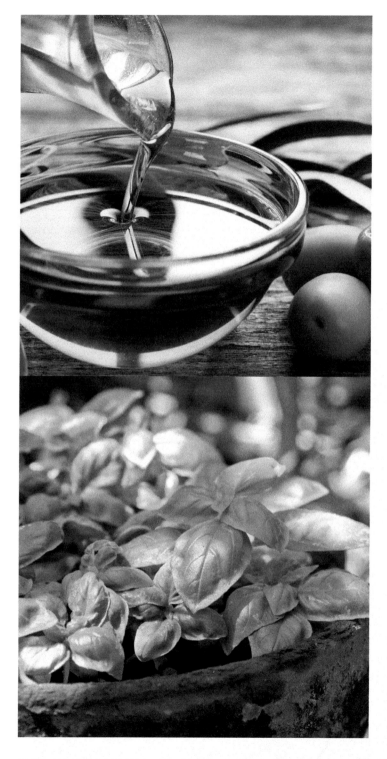

You'll notice from the labels around the 'plate', our guide is very much about eating whole foods – ones that haven't been processed to within an inch of their lives!

Processing can really damage foods. It also breaks down chains of carbohydrates, so they're converted to blood sugar much more quickly in our bodies. And of course, long-term, high levels of blood sugar leads to a lack of metabolic flexibility, insulin-resistance and type 2 diabetes.

Fats & oils

It's not easy to see the oils and fats in our plate, but we recommend generous use of healthy fats – there'll also be quite a bit in some of the animal products too if you eat them. We go into this a bit further on, but around 50-60% of the energy value of this plate will come from fats, although it looks like only 10% by weight. This is very different from what most government guidelines say because, bottom line, it's hard to be healthy without enough fat in your diet.

Spread your healthy fats through cooking, salad and veg dressings, avocados, nuts, some seeds and animal products if you eat them.

Protein sources

When we talk about 25% protein-rich foods, this doesn't mean that's the protein level in the food. Most of any fresh, animal protein source, like meat or fish, is actually water, so maybe around 20% protein by weight. But you also need to factor in veg proteins, like legumes from the pea, bean and lentil family that are rich sources.

Top tip! Slow cook your legumes to neutralise the lectins – a plant's natural pesticide that it uses to defend itself from insect pests in particular. That's why a traditional Indian dahl is often slow-cooked for around 6 h. A useful short cut if you don't have time is a pressure cooker, especially if you use legumes as your key protein source.

Herbs & Spices

Get in plenty of concentrated sources of nutrients like herbs and spices, as well as herbal teas and, where needed, food supplements as well. Supplements are just another form of concentrated nutrient. Our food supply has become so simplified as it's become more and more globalised and industrialised that many suffer the effects of insufficient nutrient diversity. That's why we give these concentrated nutrients their own slice of the plate!

Grains

You might wonder why we've left grains to last when governments and a large part of the food industry are telling us grains are our staple food. Well, the Food4health guide – now used by a lot of nutritional practitioners – says it differently. For us – your non-starchy veg is your staple, not your grains. Grains can be an important source of fibre, as well as certain vitamins and minerals, but we can also get all these micronutrients and fibres from other food sources.

Most grains are energy dense, but not nutrient dense. That means they give you lots of calories but not a whole lot else, especially if they're highly refined or processed. As grains are carbs, a lot of those calories break down to sugars in your body and then you're in danger of derailing your metabolic flexibility. No matter what you may have been told, you can get plenty of energy from your veg as plant foods are carbs too! Many grains also contain gluten, which affects a large part of the population adversely.

So, make grains only a small part of your diet, keep them whole and choose gluten-free versions like buckwheat, oats, millet, teff, quinoa, rice or sorghum where you can.

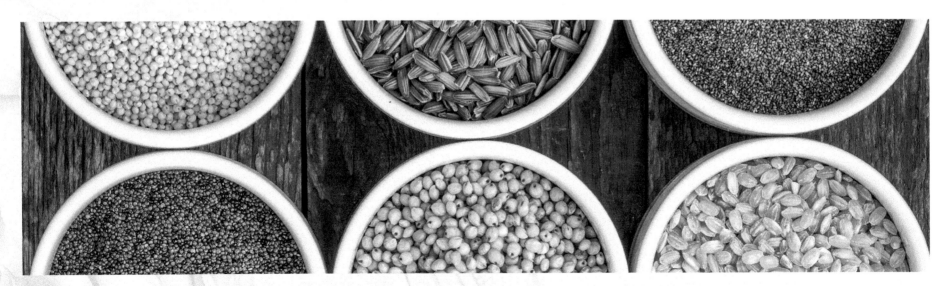

©2022 ALLIANCE FOR NATURAL HEALTH INTERNATIONAL

And here is our Food4Kids 'plate' (find out more on page 95).

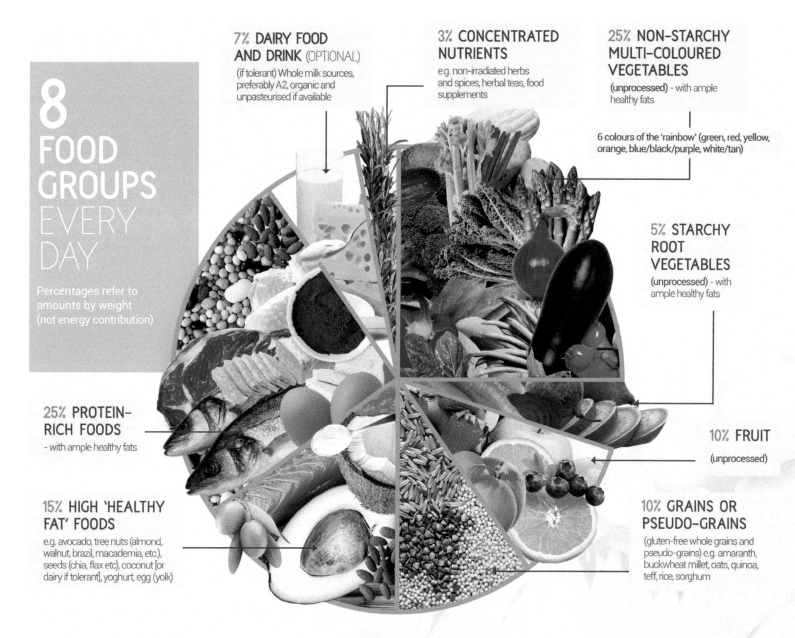

8 FOOD GROUPS EVERY DAY

Percentages refer to amounts by weight (not energy contribution)

7% DAIRY FOOD AND DRINK (OPTIONAL)

(if tolerant) Whole milk sources, preferably A2, organic and unpasteurised if available

3% CONCENTRATED NUTRIENTS

e.g. non-irradiated herbs and spices, herbal teas, food supplements

25% NON-STARCHY MULTI-COLOURED VEGETABLES

(unprocessed) - with ample healthy fats

6 colours of the 'rainbow' (green, red, yellow, orange, blue/black/purple, white/tan)

5% STARCHY ROOT VEGETABLES

(unprocessed) - with ample healthy fats

25% PROTEIN-RICH FOODS

- with ample healthy fats

15% HIGH 'HEALTHY FAT' FOODS

e.g. avocado, tree nuts (almond, walnut, brazil, macademia, etc.), seeds (chia, flax etc), coconut [or dairy if tolerant], yoghurt, egg (yolk)

10% FRUIT

(unprocessed)

10% GRAINS OR PSEUDO-GRAINS

(gluten-free whole grains and pseudo-grains) e.g. amaranth, buckwheat millet, oats, quinoa, teff, rice, sorghum

FOOD4KIDS GUIDELINES

The 10 key Food4Health guidelines

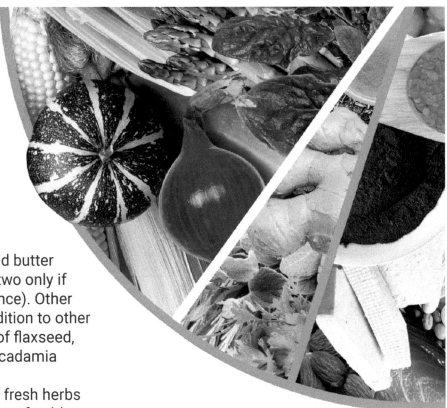

1. Macronutrient contribution by energy (kcal or kJ) should be approximately 20% protein (4 kcal/g), 25% carbohydrates (4 kcal/g) and 55% fats (9 kcal/g) - based on daily 'plate' illustrated above

2. Minimise consumption of highly processed foods and avoid all refined carbohydrates

3. Consume plenty of fresh, raw or lightly cooked plant foods (vegetables and fruit, in a roughly 4:1 ratio) that include all 6 colours of the 'rainbow' each day (green, red, yellow, orange, blue/black/purple, white/tan/brown)

4. Avoid high-temperature cooking methods (frying, grilling, BBQ), unless brief. Minimise heat-damage to proteins, fats, vegetables, starches and other carbs by using slow cooking methods

5. Healthy fats for cooking include virgin coconut oil, unfiltered extra virgin olive oil, virgin avocado oil, safflower oil, and butter or ghee (the latter two only if no lactose intolerance). Other healthy fats for addition to other foods include oils of flaxseed, hempseed and macadamia

6. Consume plenty of fresh herbs and non-irradiated, preferably organic, spices, along with herbal teas (with real herbs/spices, not flavourings)

7. Avoid snacking and try to maintain 5 or more hours between meals

8. Consume at least 1.5 litres of spring or filtered water daily between meals (more if exercising intensively)

9. Avoid all foods which trigger sensitivity, intolerance or allergy

10. Seek advice from a qualified and experienced nutritional health professional on the most appropriate concentrated sources of nutrients, herbal teas and/or supplements (concentrated sources of nutrients)

©2022 ALLIANCE FOR NATURAL HEALTH INTERNATIONAL

A bit of number crunching

For those of you who want to understand more about the numbers, here goes...

Our guideline 'plate' is based on the fresh weight of the food, as against most other food guidelines that refer to the relative energy contribution of each macronutrient, namely protein, fats and carbs.

In essence, our plate looks like this **by weight:**

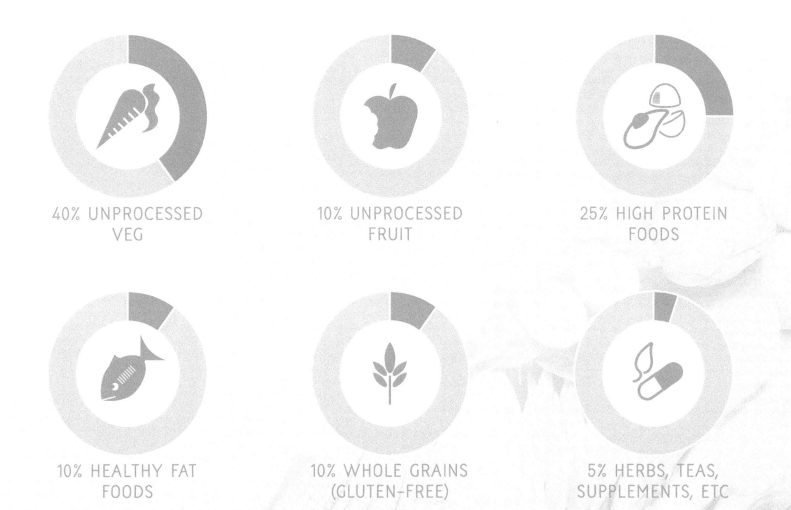

40% UNPROCESSED VEG

10% UNPROCESSED FRUIT

25% HIGH PROTEIN FOODS

10% HEALTHY FAT FOODS

10% WHOLE GRAINS (GLUTEN-FREE)

5% HERBS, TEAS, SUPPLEMENTS, ETC

©2022 ALLIANCE FOR NATURAL HEALTH INTERNATIONAL

We've factored in various food combinations that fit this pattern and a typical macronutrient composition—still **by weight**—looks something like this:

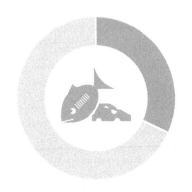

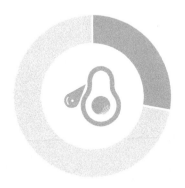

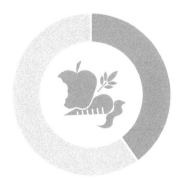

32% PROTEIN-BASED FOODS, MAINLY FROM MEATS (WHERE PRESENT), VEG, NUTS/SEEDS, CHEESE/DAIRY (WHERE PRESENT), ETC.

28% HEALTHY FAT-BASED FOODS, MAINLY FROM OILS, SEEDS, NUTS, OILY FRUITS LIKE AVOCADO, AND FROM MEATS (WHERE PRESENT)

40% CARBOHYDRATE-BASED FOODS, MAINLY FROM VEG, FRUITS AND GRAINS (WHERE PRESENT)

Now, if you look at the above ratios in terms of their energy contribution you have to take into account the energy derived from each macronutrient based on the accepted premise that each gram of protein and carb yields 4 kcal (calories) respectively, and fat yields a whopping 9 kcal per gram.

This simple premise combined with the (misplaced) view that it is just caloric excess that is driving the obesity epidemic inspires governments to push low fat diets.

Implicit within this obsession to drive the public to consume fewer calories are two more, even more deeply misplaced assumptions:

a) that all calories behave in similar ways in each person's body and

b) that the quality of the food and other nutrients contained within a given calorie of food are identical.

©2022 ALLIANCE FOR NATURAL HEALTH INTERNATIONAL

Anyway, looking again at the macronutrient ratios for the Food4Health guideline 'plate', but now from an **energy contribution** viewpoint, we end up with roughly the following ratios:

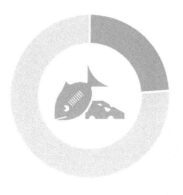

20% PROTEIN

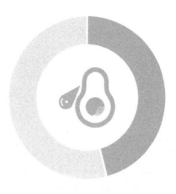

50% FAT

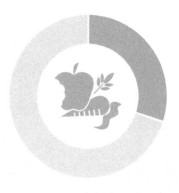

30% CARBOHYDRATE

But these are just our starting ratios to help you transition from where you might be, to a more evolutionary-rationale energy composition. You can flex your ratios as necessary. Particularly by increasing the relative amounts of healthy fats and decreasing complex carbs. Vegans will also tend to have to cope with lower protein intakes than omnivores and flexitarians.

If you are extremely active, for example, you might end up benefiting from closer to 70% of your energy from fats. But, to do that you need to be ketoadapted, highly active and have no insurmountable genetic impairments in your ability to metabolise fats.

FOOD IS INFORMATION

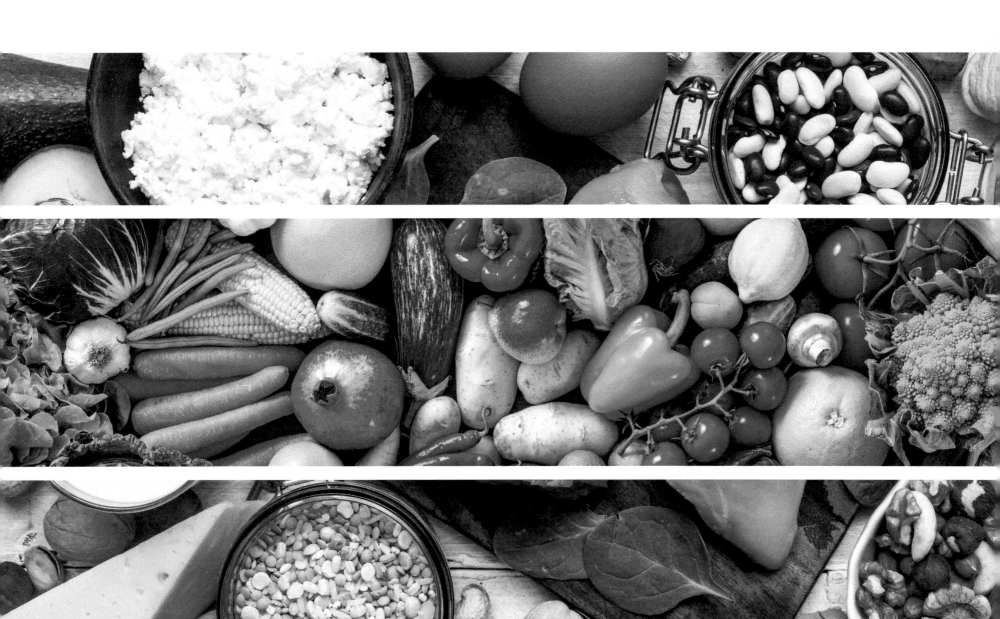

When it comes to food, we ignore our genes and evolutionary history at our peril. As well as being a carrier for energy, food is a profound source of biochemical information that needs to communicate in a language that our genes recognise and can interpret. While we've had the odd upgrade here and there, the main genetic blueprint we're running is a Paleolithic one. That's one of the reasons it's struggling to cope with the incredibly rapid changes in our food supply since agriculture became industrialised. Changes that include much more processing (think additives, preservatives, artificial sweeteners), GMOs, a massively simplified diet as well as one that is frequently sterile. Because of this, we modern humans are at risk of losing a good deal of our ancestral vigour!

Food literally changes the way our genes express. Far from being set or static, our genes are constantly being turned on or off - amplified or silenced. And this process is what dramatically affects our response to changes in our environment. Our health depends on our ability to adapt, to become resilient in the face of change.

You may have heard the term 'epigenetics', which refers to the effects of diet, lifestyle and environmental factors on our genetic expression. But the exciting bit of this is that changes in the expression of our DNA towards either health or disease are significantly under our direct control. This is because of the power of the foods we eat, the amount of activity we engage in, how we manage our stress and how much sleep we get to shunt our gene expression in a certain direction.

When we make the right food choices to inform healthful gene expression we open up to a new world of health and healing with metabolic flexibility at its core. It's very hard for disease to flourish in a resilient, vital body that adapts to change easily — and is in a 'flexi-keto' state. It's why we're still here as a species and it's how we find the road back to health again.

 ©2022 ALLIANCE FOR NATURAL HEALTH INTERNATIONAL

FOOD IS
INFORMATION

A healthy, diverse diet contains a multitude of components that provide the plethora of interacting biochemical pathways the information they need to regulate the 12 key body systems

BODY SYSTEMS

BODY SYSTEM NAME	AREA OF FUNCTION
ENDOCRINE	HORMONAL
CARDIOVASCULAR	HEART AND CIRCULATION
RESPIRATORY	BREATHING/RESPIRATORY
IMMUNE	IMMUNE
NERVOUS	NERVOUS
REPRODUCTIVE/GENITAL	SEXUAL
RENAL/URINARY/EXCRETORY	DETOXIFICATION
GASTROINTESTINAL	DIGESTIVE
MUSCULAR	MUSCULAR
SKELETAL	BONES AND JOINTS
INTEGUMENTAL	SKIN, HAIR AND NAILS
OPTHALMOLOGICAL	VISUAL/EYE

ANH-Intl's **Food4Health** Guidelines for adults and **Food4Kids** Guidelines for young children, will help you make better choices in what, when and how you eat!

"The most profound revelation for me in my own healing journey back from autoimmune thyroid disease was truly understanding how much influence my nutrition and life choices have over my genes. This was - and still is - profoundly empowering for me. It's enabled me to stick to my regime because it's given me my health and vitality back. Priceless."

- Meleni Aldridge BSc NutrMed Dip cPNI

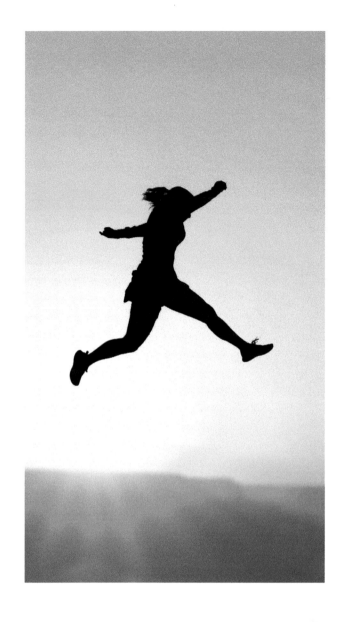

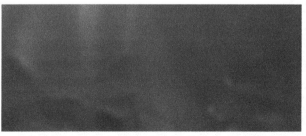

Metabolic flexibility and resilience - markers of health

Our genetic and epigenetic backgrounds, as well as our levels of activity, stress and lifestyles, all demand different food compositions. No one should eat the same composition of foods and macronutrients (protein, fats and carbs) every day, day in day out. That's because our activity pattern, stress and other elements of our lifestyle are, or should be, in a continuous state of flux.

This brings us to two key points: metabolic flexibility and resilience. These are the real markers of health. Metabolic flexibility refers to the capacities to adapt to, and burn (oxidise), whichever fuel is available. Someone who has developed metabolic flexibility — i.e. has become 'flexi-keto' adapted — can therefore handle a more variable diet and can burn fats effectively, these being the richest source of energy for the body.

Physiological resilience refers to your ability to respond to and recover from physiological, metabolic, immunological or lifestyle stress. Someone who is resilient, is someone who can regain equilibrium — or homeostasis — more quickly than someone who may be free from clinical symptoms of disease, but ultimately, lacks this supreme level of vibrant, resilient, and ultimately, adaptive health.

There are a few principles that are common among those who obtain this state of metabolic flexibility and resilience. These include:

- They are keto-adapted and are able to readily burn fats for fuel

- They regularly practice caloric restriction through fasting between meals. This is quite different from just eating fewer calories every day, but still little and often!

- They are physically active

- Their diet is anti-inflammatory and loaded with phytonutrients from the 6 main colour groups of the phytonutrient spectrum

- The bulk of their diet, in terms of its energy contribution, does not come from carbohydrates - wholegrain or otherwise!

- They show no signs of metabolic syndrome or insulin resistance, either in muscles or in other tissues and therefore have ideal or near-ideal body compositions (muscle/adipose/visceral fat ratios)

- They have modified their nutritional intake, eating habits and lifestyle in such a way as to largely offset any disadvantageous genetic limitations they may carry

- Their diet and activity levels create psycho-emotional flexibility as well, meaning more emotional balance – and yes, happiness too!

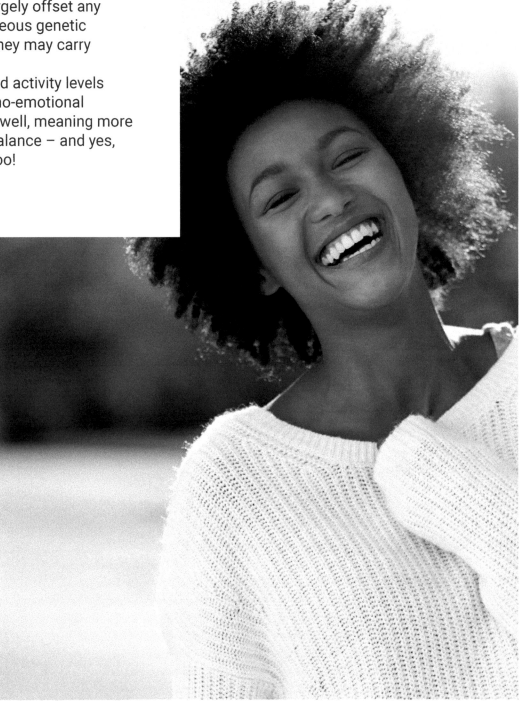

©2022 ALLIANCE FOR NATURAL HEALTH INTERNATIONAL

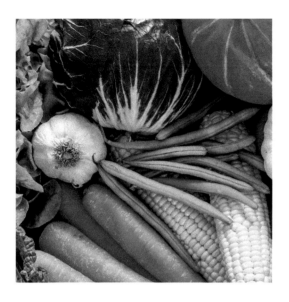

It's not just about what's on your plate

How and when you eat has a huge impact on your health. This includes how you prepare your food, how you chew it, when you eat, how long you leave between meals, along with your genetic background, lifestyle, physical activity and nutritional needs. All are crucial to deciding how the food will interact with your metabolism.

But if there's one additional message specific to nutrition that is stronger than any other, we'd argue it is the need to fast regularly. That means daily. And the easiest way of doing this is to try to fast 12 hours overnight and 5 hours between meals. This has been a central plank to the Metabolic Balance programme that has helped many tens of thousands to reset their metabolism and endocrine system, helping people to emerge from insulin resistance, pre-diabetes, metabolic syndrome and even type 2 diabetes. Eating little and often, as recommended by the vast bulk of dietitians, simply pushes people into insulin resistance and a downward spiral of associated metabolic diseases that now plague our society.

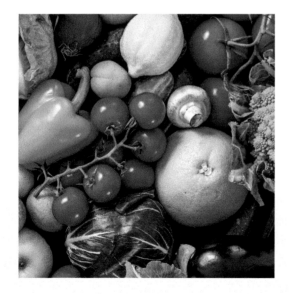

Food as 'fuel': storing and using energy (the science bit!)

If you're keen on living naturally and minimising your recourse to drugs for as long as possible, it's very important to understand something about the ways in which we burn food as fuel – and how we store our fuels. Doing this right will help you to become — or stay — lean and fit, while reducing your reliance on the healthcare system and especially pharmaceutical medicines. It's about helping you to take back control of your health, in the event you might have already handed that responsibility to someone else, or are concerned that, later in life, that responsibility may be wrested from you.

Most people, with the support of government guidelines, consume a balance of too many carbs and not enough fats. We now understand that consuming little fat and lots of carbs, especially refined ones, and even consuming too much protein, stops you from becoming what we call 'keto-adapted' (an efficient fat burner). In a high-fat nutshell, the dormancy of the fat burning capacity, a condition facing millions, is a major, and often unspoken, contributor to the present obesity epidemic and chronic disease spiral.

How do you burn your fuel?

Over millennia, our bodies have developed very intelligent systems for turning the food we eat into the energy we need to run all of our internal metabolism, build new DNA and cells, run our brains and immune systems (that are among the two biggest energy sinks we have), digest our food — and all of that (and much more) before we even become active and fuel our mitochondria (more on these as you read on) and muscles!

Let's look at carbs first, given that many dietitians and public health authorities still tell us they should represent the primary source of our energy.

Carbs are basically long chains, simple or complex, of glucose. We get energy out of glucose (a 6-carbon sugar) by splitting each molecule into two 3-carbon sugars. We refer to this process as glycolysis which literally means 'sugar splitting'. In the absence of oxygen, in other words during anaerobic glycolysis, every molecule of glucose generates, via a series of enzyme-controlled steps, only very limited amounts of energy in the form of two molecules of ATP (adenosine triphosphate). But it also produces two molecules of pyruvic acid (pyruvate).

> ANAEROBIC GLYCOLYSIS OF EACH GLUCOSE MOLECULE YIELDS JUST TWO ATP MOLECULES

Still in the absence of oxygen, such as when you're exercising for extended periods close to your maximum limit, you start to ferment this pyruvate, yielding lactic acid (**Fig. 1**). Interestingly, even when the skeletal muscles in your arms and legs are secreting this lactate, a healthy heart can still function using the aerobic glycolytic pathway (see **Fig. 1**) because, being so filled with blood, it has an extraordinary ability to metabolise the lactate into carbon dioxide.

While ATP is the primary fuel used for most reactions in the body most of the time, this small amount of energy from anaerobic glycolysis is used mainly to produce energy carriers like NADH and FADH2.

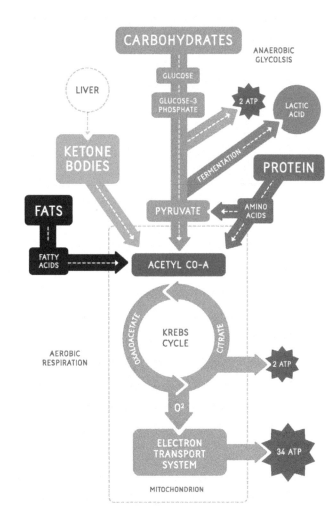

Figure 1. Key anaerobic and aerobic pathways for cellular respiration of macronutrients

 ©2022 ALLIANCE FOR NATURAL HEALTH INTERNATIONAL

Let's not forget, we need a lot of ATP, in the order of half or more of your body weight's worth daily! Some of this we get from our food, some we get by recycling ATP. We get energy from ATP by breaking the high-energy bond in the molecule when one of its phosphorus groups is enzymatically cleaved from it so forming ADP (adenosine diphosphate). We can then use energy from our food, produced in the mitochondria, to convert the ADP back to ATP.

Put oxygen into the equation and it's a very different story. If you are replete with oxygen, and therefore are not exercising near your limit and exceeding your lactate threshold, you get to burn your carbs via the aerobic glycolysis pathway. Here, the pyruvate is used, following its conversion to acetyl co-enzyme A (often referred to as acetyl-coA), a key substrate for the Krebs (citric acid) cycle in the energy-generating factories we have in cells, especially muscle cells, called mitochondria. You may only get 2 ATP molecules directly from Krebs (also used mainly to generate energy carriers), but Krebs metabolites, along with various cofactors including coenzyme Q10, then set off the proton gradient that

yields the bulk of mitochondrial energy in the electron transport system (ETS). This is the main way we get energy from carbs, proteins and fats. And when we oxidise glucose, we get a somewhat impressive 34 molecules of ATP for each molecule of glucose.

Another point is that we can store glucose, but not very much of it.

> **AEROBIC GLYCOLYSIS OF EACH GLUCOSE MOLECULE YIELDS AN ADDITIONAL 34 ATP MOLECULES**

We do this in the form of glycogen. We can store around 100 grams of glycogen in the liver and about 400 grams in the muscles. Most people have burned this up after around 90 mins of strenuous activity in the absence of other fuel.

Now, what about proteins and fats?

> **JUST ONE MOLECULE OF A FATTY ACID YIELDS A STUNNING 129 ATP MOLECULES**

Oxidation of proteins and fats

These also get oxidised to form energy in the form of ATP. What is key to appreciate is that the oxidation of proteins and fats, as seen in Figure 1, also converge on the Krebs cycle. In the case of proteins, they must be oxidised to their constituent amino acids (of which there are 20 in total), and have their nitrogen removed in order to become substrates that are used directly or indirectly in the Krebs cycle. These reactions that allow inter-conversion between amino acids and energy substrates are called transamination and deamination reactions. Glutamate is also a critical player because it is the key transporter of amino acids in the blood, while exerting other key functions such as helping to maintain integrity of the intestinal lining and supporting the immune system and kidneys.

Gram for gram protein yields about the same amount of energy as carbohydrates. That's one of the reasons food labelling laws require that manufacturers stipulate that 4 calories (kcal) are yielded for every gram of carb or protein contained in a food. Actually, that's only the case if you both absorb and oxidise the fuel fully. The latter is usually determined on a lab bench using a bomb calorimeter - not in a body! The problem is many people don't digest, absorb or oxidise their fuels fully because of one or more impairments, these being genetic or physiological.

We've left the best to last! Fats yield energy from oxidation too and the products of oxidation, just like carbs and protein, converge on the Krebs cycle. Fats are broken down to their constituent fatty acids via what's called the beta-oxidation pathway, mainly in the liver. They then yield the common denominator acetyl-coA via 4 reactions that occur again in the mitochondria (and peroxisomes), mainly in the liver and muscles.

If you take just one molecule of a fatty acid, say palmitate, you can generate a stunning theoretical yield of 129 ATP molecules using the beta-oxidation pathway! This makes even the 34 ATP yield from aerobic glycolysis from a glucose molecule look somewhat paltry.

MITOCHONDRIA

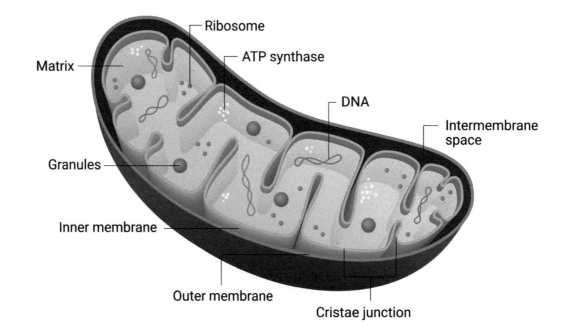

Matrix

Ribosome

ATP synthase

DNA

Intermembrane space

Granules

Inner membrane

Outer membrane

Cristae junction

©2022 ALLIANCE FOR NATURAL HEALTH INTERNATIONAL

Nutritional ketosis

But that's not all. If the amount of carbohydrate consumed is limited, especially while the energy requirement is increased (ie. as a result of exercise), more acetyl-coA will be produced from the beta-oxidation (burning/processing) of fatty acids. If there is more than is required to meet the energy needs of an individual, this excess acetyl-coA will be shunted into another process called ketogenesis, that yields ketone bodies (acetoacetate, β-hydroxybutyrate and acetone). These then become an additional metabolic fuel.

From an evolutionary perspective, this pathway has been vital to human success and is clear evidence for just how well we are adapted to starvation and what we now think of as 'intermittent fasting' (ie. NOT three meals a day with snacks in between). Without carbs, proteins and fats from our food, in other words during starvation, we can actually use ketone bodies produced by beta-oxidation of our own fat deposits as our primary fuel for vital organs such as the brain and heart. You literally burn fat in your sleep!

For a long time, scientists and doctors thought of ketosis, the process that generates ketone bodies, as a bad thing. That's because it was associated with either starvation, or uncontrolled diabetics, who can develop serious and life-threatening diabetic ketoacidosis. When ketone bodies develop excessively in the body you can smell a strong, characteristic fruity, pear drop smell on the breath. This is the result of high levels of acetone being produced.

As shown by Drs Jeff Volek and Steve Phinney in their bestselling book, *The Art and Science of Low Carb Living*, healthy, nutritional ketosis is established when serum (blood) concentrations of ketone bodies are in the range 0.5-3.0 mM. This is what they refer to as the "optimal ketone zone" and can be achieved with a low carb, relatively high fat, ketogenic diet, such as that consumed when you follow the Food4Health guideline 'plate'.

Starvation ketosis and ketoacidosis don't occur until levels of ketone bodies are around 3 to 20 times greater than this. You can now measure your level of nutritional ketosis simply and easily through urine, blood or more recently, breath testing using a Ketone Meter.

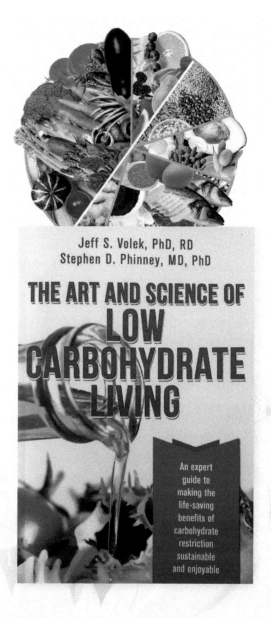

Jeff S. Volek, PhD, RD
Stephen D. Phinney, MD, PhD

THE ART AND SCIENCE OF LOW CARBOHYDRATE LIVING

An expert guide to making the life-saving benefits of carbohydrate restriction sustainable and enjoyable

©2022 ALLIANCE FOR NATURAL HEALTH INTERNATIONAL

As far as storage and use of proteins and fats are concerned, if we don't have enough carbs in our body, and we haven't adapted to burning fats because we have not yet adapted to switching to the fatty acid-burning beta-oxidation pathway, we can start burning protein, especially in muscles. This is never a good thing, especially if you're interested in improving your lean muscle mass and being physically very active.

We're all aware of how readily we store energy as fat. We also know that the main reason people get fat is not from eating too much fat, but by eating too little —and too much carbohydrate. Fat can exist in many forms and is stored in different ways and places including beneath the skin (as adipose tissue) or around the organs (as visceral fat). Generally, the latter is the most dangerous and needn't be that visible, hence recent concerns about the risk of being 'skinny fat' ie. thin on the outside, fat on the inside. This, once again, is an increasingly common predicament triggered by low fat recommendations which have led to dependence on and addiction to refined carbs from soft drinks, white bread and other ultra-processed, high glycaemic foods.

A bit of brown adipose tissue (BAT) or brown fat, on the other hand, is the healthiest fat to lay down. It becomes a key fuel if you are both keto-adapted and want the stamina of an endurance athlete.

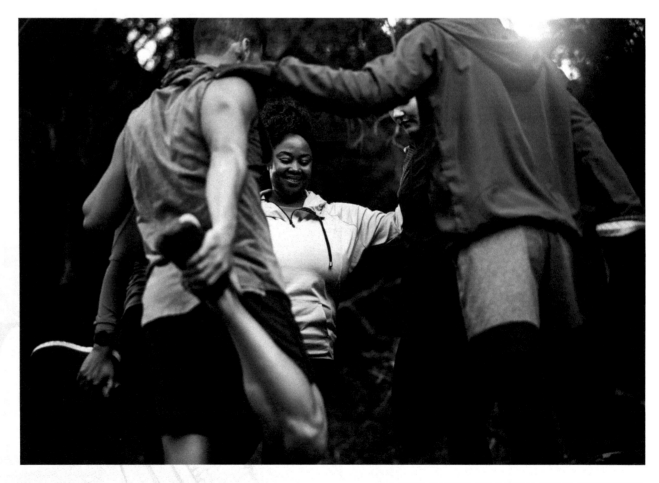

©2022 ALLIANCE FOR NATURAL HEALTH INTERNATIONAL

How physical activity fits into the picture

We've had a look so far at how the body uses different types of fuel. But physical activity and exercise has a huge bearing on how this happens. In essence, the body is able to use one of three different energy systems while you exercise.

If you exercise extremely vigorously for a few seconds, such as when you break into a sprint or you trigger your fight or flight response, you don't use ATP from cellular respiration. Instead, you rely on producing ATP, the universal fuel, from creatine phosphate of which you have very limited reserves in muscles. This is called the phosphagen, creatine phosphate or phosphocreatine system. Its plusses are that it makes energy instantly. Its downside is it doesn't make very much. That's why nearly everyone can do three or four press-ups, but some struggle to do more. The phosphagen system was there originally to allow us to sprint from sabre-toothed tigers.

The second energy system is the anaerobic glycolysis pathway we discussed earlier (Fig 1). It's about making energy from glucose in the absence of oxygen. It can't be sustained for more than about 5 minutes or so before the lactic acid accumulates excessively. Cramp is one outcome of being anaerobic too long.

The third system is the key one for long-term energy use. It's the aerobic pathway that lets us burn any of the three major macronutrient fuels. But it's the fats that are both the cleanest burning and, as we've seen above, yield by far the most energy. That's why people are waking up to easy-access fatty fuels like coconut oil, a very rich source of medium-chain triglycerides.

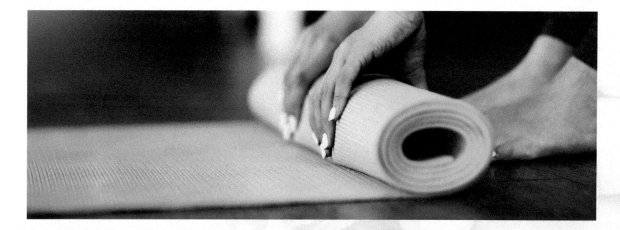

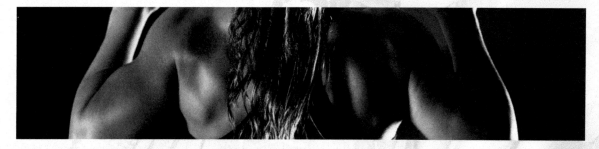

12 steps to transition
from being a carb burner to a fat burner

The ease with which you can shift from being primarily reliant on carb burning, as compared to being a keto-adapted, fat burner, varies considerably in people.

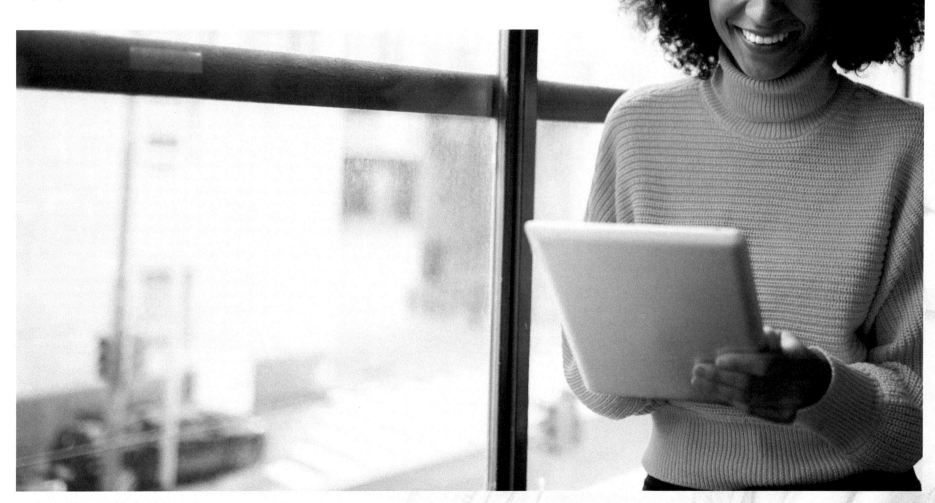

Genetics and psychology are two big factors affecting this. But assuming all things are even and that impediments to significantly changing your lifestyle are absent, here are 12 safe and simple steps you can take that will often have a dramatic effect on your transition:

1. Start eating according to the Food4Health guidelines and cut out or radically minimise grains and starchy carbs. Whilst you do this, also avoid snacks of any type between meals, especially ones that are rich in simple carbs (it's okay to drink water)

2. Maintain a 12-hour overnight fast on at least 5 days a week, but longer if you can. Fifteen - 18 hours is optimal, but it may take you 6-8 weeks to achieve this with ease

3. Leave at least 5 hours between meals or any form of food intake to allow your gastrointestinal tract to rest, lower inflammation and allow your insulin to come back to baseline again

4. Engage in high intensity physical activity (if your level of fitness permits it) for short periods (say 15 to 45 minutes) around twice weekly. This is often best carried out in the form of high intensity interval training (HIIT)

5. Engage in some periods—say three times a week—of longer, lower intensity endurance exercise (in excess of 1.5 hours on each occasion) to help the body move into beta-oxidation of fats after muscle and liver glycogen has been depleted. For most people, this can be done at around 55-75% of your maximal heart rate (meaning you can still speak in sentences without being breathless). Avoid popping energy gels or other sources of carbohydrate during these sessions as they will switch off fat burning

6. Support the health of your mitochondria (the energy factories in your cells), and stimulate the creation of more, by doing the '3-min Anytime Anywhere HIIT' routine at least once a day, but 3 x for maximum effect

7. Consume at least 25g of protein and perhaps 5g of glutamine and 5g of branched-chain amino acids within a 30-minute window following completion of intense exercise to help your muscles to recover

8. Stretch those muscles that have been worked carefully after bouts of intense and extended exercise

9. Rest sufficiently between bouts of exercise, so that your muscles can rebuild and compensate following the damage caused by the exercise. This in turn acts as a trigger to build bigger, stronger and leaner muscle

10. Be honest about your needs around stress and take steps to manage it. Stress derails our health because it affects so many systems. Incorporate some simple mindfulness and breathing techniques into your day to calm your sympathetic nervous system and transform 'fight & flight' into 'rest & digest'

©2022 ALLIANCE FOR NATURAL HEALTH INTERNATIONAL

11. Prioritise your sleep and make sure you get 6-8 hours of good quality sleep a night in a pitch-dark room. Your body can't rejuvenate, regenerate or heal when you scrimp on sleep!

12. Plan for health. Getting the balance between your nutritional intake and your physical activity regime right is both an art and a science. It's also highly individual, given variations in genetics, aptitude, opportunity and environment, amongst other factors. Keeping a food and training diary can be very helpful where you note how you *feel* after food and activity because your body is an accurate barometer.

Integrating these approaches into your life is the best way of experiencing a very high level of vital health. However, that's easier said than done given time and other constraints that apply to so many of us.

The point is, doing **something** right is always better than doing nothing right!

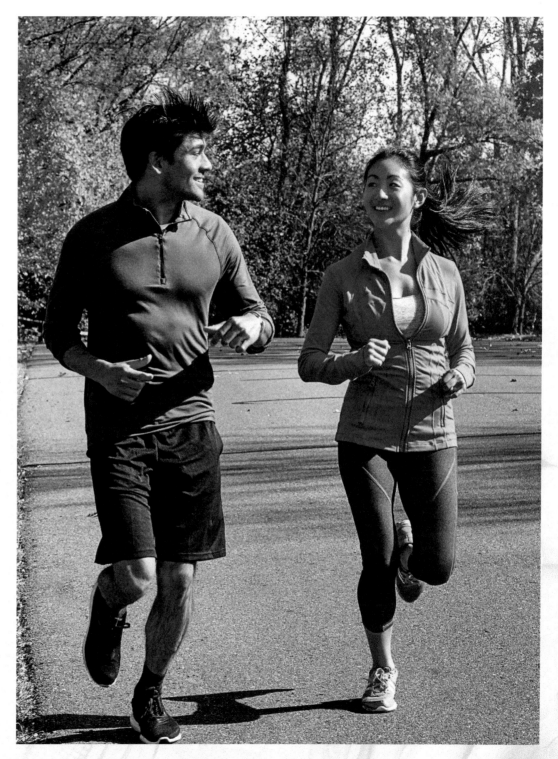

Calorie restriction & intermittent fasting - encoded in our evolutionary blueprint

Points 1 to 3 in the previous section are so critical to re-tuning your metabolism that we've devoted an entire section to discussing why. Whilst the jury may still be out on the specifics of the diets of our paleolithic ancestors, one thing is certain, early *Homo sapiens sapiens* didn't have the luxury of kitchens with well-stocked refrigerators!

Our ancestors definitely had to expend energy to feed themselves and there would have been many a lean time through the last 200,000 years. But despite the lean times and the effort required to find food in plenty of inhospitable environments, our species has survived and flourished. Therein lies a clue. Perhaps Nature factored calorie restriction and exercise into our basic blueprint? And perhaps in doing so, She turned a potential negative to a positive? It's more than interesting that, malnutrition aside, those of our species that don't have access to 'food on tap', generally live longer, healthier and happier lives. And they certainly don't suffer the long list of diseases common to those of the species with well-stocked kitchens.

Our genetic blueprint

There have been over 2,000 papers in the last ten years looking at the effects of calorie restriction on everything from single-celled organisms to primates. The general conclusion: longer, healthier lifespans, enhanced performance and optimised weight. It's known that calorie restriction affects key pathways in the body that regulate metabolism, cell growth and cell proliferation. For instance, restricting the amount of calories you eat is able to deactivate the nutrient-sensing mTOR pathway, which slows down aging and prevents age-related diseases such as type II diabetes; it can also regulate insulin levels and insulin-like growth factors necessary for blood sugar control and cell growth, to name but two. When these and other metabolic pathways become disturbed, the result is, unfortunately, obesity, shorter lifespans and increased incidence of chronic disease.

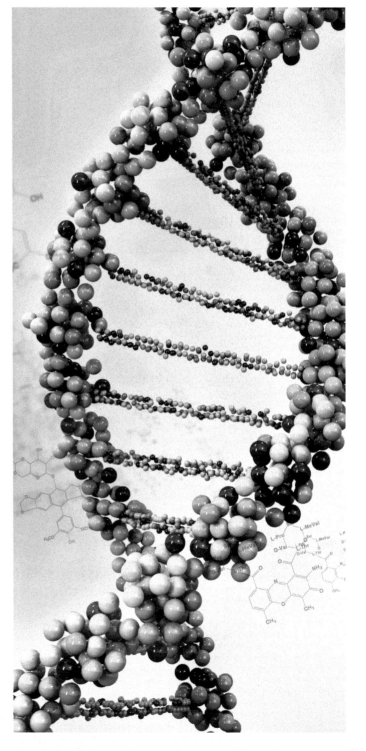

©2022 ALLIANCE FOR NATURAL HEALTH INTERNATIONAL

Coming back to our basic genetic blueprint as *Homo sapiens sapiens*, as we've already discussed, maintaining health is all about maintaining metabolic flexibility. In other words, the ability to provide sufficient energy for our bodies to perform, but not so much that we need to start storing the excess as fat and creating disease. The excess being the curse, rather than the luxury, of our modern world — the 'Well-Stocked Kitchen Syndrome'.

Starving for better health

Our bodies are perfectly adapted to periods of starvation and have developed a number of systems for maintaining sufficient energy for the brain, immune system and performance. Researcher, Mikhail Blagosklonny explains that to feed the brain during non-malnutrition starvation (ie. intermittent fasting), the liver produces glucose from protein building blocks, amino acids, (gluconeogenesis) and ketones from fatty acids (ketogenesis). Fat cells (adipocytes) need to release the fatty acids to fuel the ketogenesis and secretion of insulin by the pancreas is therefore decreased to enable the liver to carry out these specific functions. The key

noticeable metabolic alterations arising from restricting calories are that your alternate energy pathways kick in (gluconeogenesis, ketogenesis), your insulin levels lower and, if you need it, you lose body fat as you burn it for energy.

In short, our body has been made to split its own proteins and fats to make energy—becoming metabolically flexible—rather than needing to consume huge amounts of calories for energy. Remember the old adage; 'use it before you lose it'? Well, it's the over consumption of calories (particularly empty carbohydrate calories) that disables our metabolic flexibility in the first place, hinders our fat burning potential and prevents us from developing resilience.

Mimicking our ancestors

When you combine calorie restriction with exercise, as our ancestors did, the many benefits include leaner bodies, better blood sugar handling (more insulin sensitivity), very low inflammation and higher levels of the fat-burning protein called adiponectin. It's also been shown that people who live like this have heart rate variability—a marker for aging and health—similar to healthy people 20 years their junior!

So, by mimicking our predecessors and eating less frequently (no snacking between meals), including regular intermittent fasting (starvation) of between 15 – 18 hours and ensuring that exercise is taken before we resume eating in our fasting window, we can regain and prime our metabolic flexibility and resilience. The results of which include extending life, delaying disease, enhancing performance (mental, emotional and physical) and optimising weight. It's really not difficult to do this if you optimise your nutrition by following the Food4Health guide.

But — a word of reassurance here for those of you who don't feel you burn fat easily or have difficulty digesting it from food. The first will get easier with time – it's perfectly normal for your body to require a little longer than average to keto-adapt. And the second issue can be helped along by taking some good quality digestive enzymes with your meal until your gastro-intestinal workings are settled and humming happily again after changing the way you eat. However, if you have a prolonged issue regarding fat digestion, please don't struggle on and do go and see a nutrition health professional. Poor fat handlers often experience a feeling of nausea when they transition to high fat diets, their gut might feel uncomfortable, and they can suffer from unpleasant smelling wind.

For many, especially regular high carb snackers, the body's fat-burning pathways can have lain dormant for decades and, just like your car engine needs specific tuning, so too does our ability to burn (beta-oxidise) fat. The ability to efficiently beta-oxidise fatty acids in our liver is a lot down to our genetic inheritance. From an evolutionary perspective, it was essential to survival because we needed to be able to cope with starvation when food couldn't be found. Somewhere down the line, though, our genetic adaptations have made some of us less adept at it than others. Men are often much better fat-burners than women because, ancestrally, they were the hunters who were physically active, and women needed the ability to store more fat to feed the next generation. A strategy that smacks of unfair gender-bias today, but one we need to work around as it's seen us through thus far!

The information in these pages takes account of these kinds of genetic difference, which is one reason you won't see fat intake recommendations here as high as other experts may recommend for classic ketogenic or even more extreme low carb/high fat diets. While a number of the genes that govern beta-oxidation have now been identified, hunting them down in an individual's genetic 'book of life' is an expensive business and one not offered by many labs making it simply not accessible to most people. Our experience over the last decade or so has shown that most people, albeit at different rates and with a certain amount of tailoring, can successfully use food to push their metabolic reset button. Such a change to our environment - caused by changing the mix of carbs, fats and protein we consume - as well as (often) reducing our eating frequency as compared with 'normal eating patterns' in most modern cultures, causes our pattern of gene expression to change. The metabolic health reset means that dormant pathways are lit up, inflammation deep inside our bodies is snuffed out and, most of the time, even the least adept fat-burner gets to burn fat — even in their sleep!

An inescapable fact is that we still share with our Palaeolithic ancestors the vast majority of the exact same genes. This means creating health and maintaining resilience today requires that we pay food and lifestyle homage to both the old and the new. Consider *RESET EATING* as a road map that allows you to chart your own individual route to destination Resilient Health.

DESTINATION
RESILIENT HEALTH ▶

©2022 ALLIANCE FOR NATURAL HEALTH INTERNATIONAL

A few points to remember when restricting your calories

- Choose organic where you can and, if you're a flexitarian, go for grass-fed beef and wild fish and meats if possible.

- 'Eat a rainbow' every day in terms of the colours you include from vegetables and fruits. Including the whole colour range daily ensures you get a good selection of phytonutrients, which also means that your antioxidant intake will be high and help you fight those ageing free radicals

- Don't overeat fruit. We have no off button (satiety) for fructose (fruit sugar) and it's very hard work for the liver to have to break it all down. Also, when the liver is busy metabolising fructose, it's not burning fat!

- Start getting used to including some exercise (at least 3-4 times per week) during one of your fasting periods. Even doing the '3-min Anytime Anywhere HIIT' session is better than doing nothing

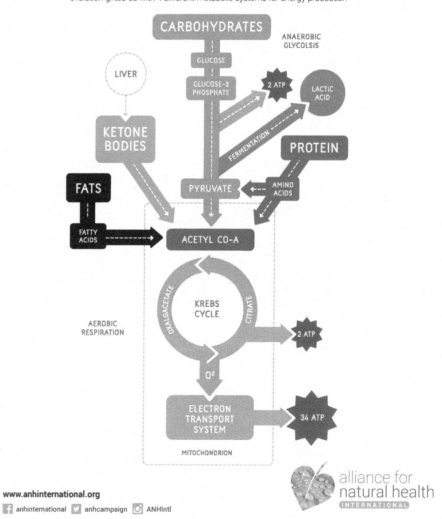

- Increase your activity levels so you are doing something daily – this includes walking up the stairs instead of taking the escalators, gardening, cleaning the house, washing the car etc. Remember we're programmed against inactivity, so get moving and mimicking our predecessors by moving before food

- As your metabolism re-tunes, it's perfectly normal to feel that you're eating too much food and you'd like to skip a meal. The timing is very individual, but don't feel anxious about dropping a meal. Your body will tell you which one. Skip it and see how you feel

- Use exercise to release more energy when you need it. It's an interesting experience to feel hungry and instead of giving in and eating straight away, go exercise and feel your body start to provide the energy you need as it burns more fat. It may take from a few weeks to a few months to get to this point, so don't force it.

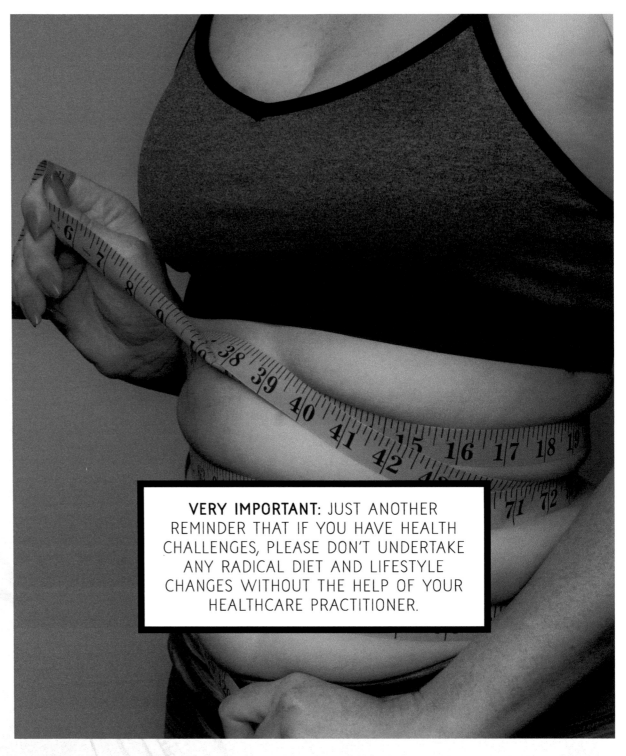

VERY IMPORTANT: JUST ANOTHER REMINDER THAT IF YOU HAVE HEALTH CHALLENGES, PLEASE DON'T UNDERTAKE ANY RADICAL DIET AND LIFESTYLE CHANGES WITHOUT THE HELP OF YOUR HEALTHCARE PRACTITIONER.

©2022 ALLIANCE FOR NATURAL HEALTH INTERNATIONAL

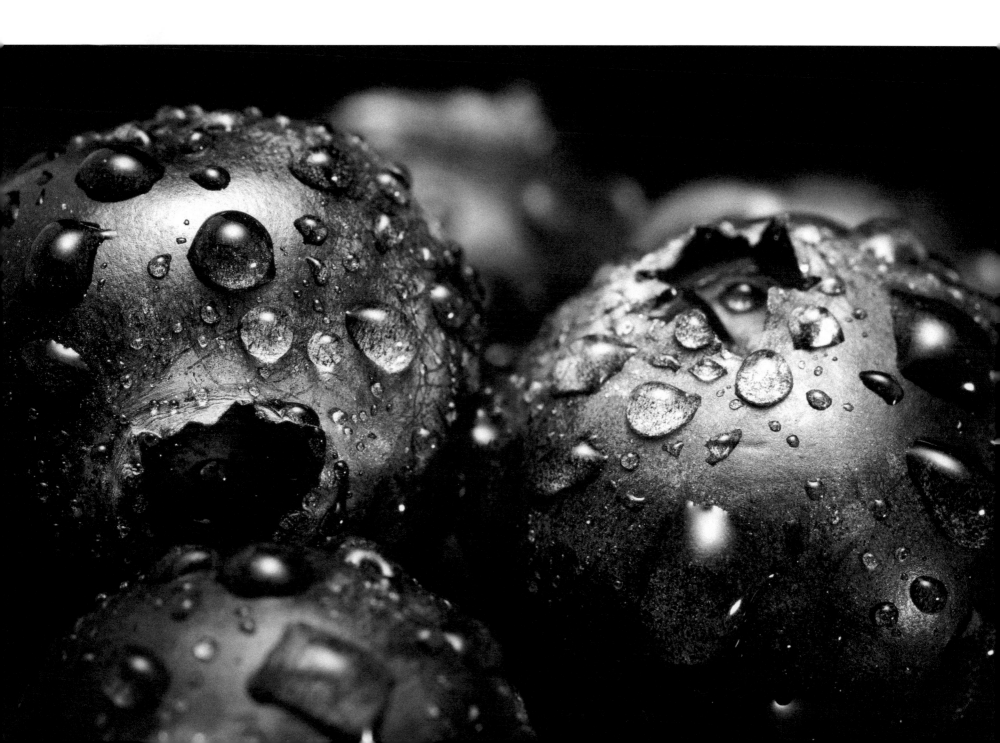

Macronutrients
1. Protein

The subject of protein is causing somewhat of a tussle right now. Whether you've read lots of media reports, have become vegan because you're passionate about the planet, subscribe to a carnivorous diet after putting your autoimmune disease into remission or are an omnivore walking an evolutionary dietary pathway, chances are you might still have some questions about protein.

Apart from the confusion arising from so many experts seemingly unable to agree (and there are some heavy hitters out there), how do you decide what you need so you can make the right food choices for You? To us, it seems as if the world of nutrition science is out to lunch on the subject of protein. Everyone appears to be fighting their corner with passion and zeal as if it's the *ONLY* way! The truth is, we're all individual and there is no one diet that will fit us all. That's why scientists who conjure up 'healthy diets' based on research and not real people tend to be off the mark with what we, as individuals, need to create optimal health.

Protein – food group, food source or energy carrier?

Protein is the collective name given to large molecules which are made up of chains of amino acids (AA). These AA chains can be hundreds or thousands in length and they are able to fold into highly complex arrangements, which gives you some idea of the complexity of proteins and an indication of their importance in our bodies. The terms peptides and polypeptides refer to the smaller chains of amino acids that make up the polymers we call proteins. If the chains are less than 30 amino acids long, we tend to refer to them as peptides, rather than proteins. Proteins not only have a host of functions within the body, they are also regarded as one of 3 essential macronutrient groups – fats and carbohydrates being the other two. We call them 'essential' because we need to ingest them in our diets – more for function than for energy – but that's why we've come to think of protein as a food group.

Having said this, all 3 macronutrients can provide the fuel (as energy carriers) for our body to sustain life. Nutritional science has long deemed, based on basic biochemistry and some rather simplistic experiments, that protein and carbs yield 4 kcal (calories) per gram and fats 9 kcal

per gram. But of course, that doesn't take into account differences in our bodies or how much energy we might expend digesting our food to extract the energy. The reality is that fat is by far the greatest energy carrier gram per gram, which is why you get more bang for your buck when you burn fats rather than carbs and one of the many reasons why the Food4Health guideline 'plate' puts you on track to keto-adapt.

Yet it's proteins that do most of the work in our cells. They're required for structure, function, regulation of our tissues and organs and particular proteins are encoded in our genes (located on our chromosones) which in turn provide vital messages or undertake specific functions in the body. If the message gets scrambled, the gene may produce a protein that has an impaired shape resulting in reduced or absent function in the body, sometimes with unpleasant consequences. That's why we've been very vocal on the subject of GMOs. Once you really understand how fundamental proteins are to life, and which genes you want switched on or off, you'd not want to mess with the natural order.

©2022 ALLIANCE FOR NATURAL HEALTH INTERNATIONAL

Coming back to amino acid chains. There are 20 different types of amino acids that combine to make a protein and it's their sequence that determines the structure and the function of that protein. Again, a reminder of how complex protein science is and how many different combinations are possible. But it's also the reason why we refer to proteins as a food source. In essence, we eat foods that contain proteins, we then chew and digest that food, the amino acid chains are broken down and the individual amino acids are released for our bodies to use.

But this process all hangs on whether we have sufficient stomach acid to break the proteins down, which is one of the reasons why taking an antacid (PPIs: proton pump inhibitors) can have such a disastrous effect on our overall health. It's also why nutritional health professionals target the gut first and foremost to restore optimal function as it's pretty much impossible to enjoy good health with a poorly functioning gut.

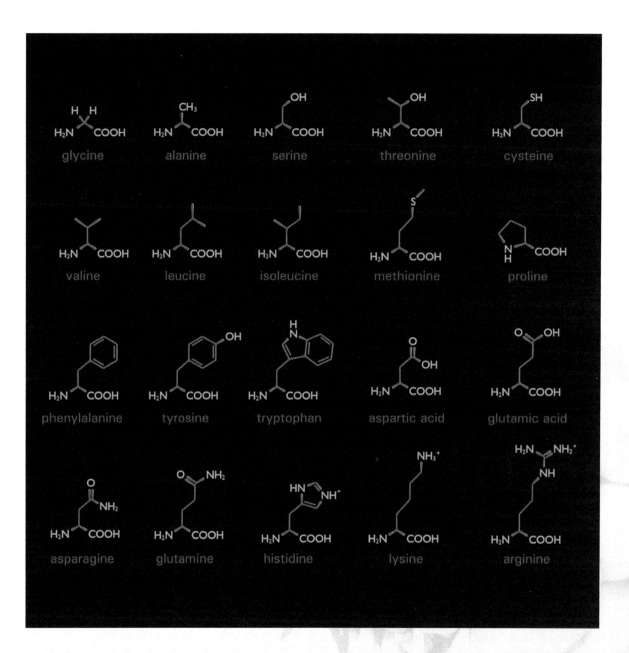

The might of amino acids

Amino acids might be small, but they're powerful and we can't survive without them. We also have to eat sufficient amounts of food containing proteins as not all amino acids are able to be made by the body.

Essential amino acids are termed such because we can't make them, they must be consumed in the diet. We can make both conditional and non-essential amino acids, but in times of enhanced need, ie. stress, illness, extreme exercise, we can run short depending instead on more coming from the diet.

As so many people are now dealing with chronic stress from modern living, as well as chronic disease and now more strenuous immune challenges, the need for good quality protein sources is central to healing, disease prevention and maintaining health.

ESSENTIAL	CONDITIONAL	NON-ESSENTIAL
Valine	Arginine	Alanine
Isoleucine	Cysteine	Asparagine
Leucine	Glutamine	Aspartic acid
Threonine	Tyrosine	
Histidine	Glycine	
Lysine	Ornithine	
Phenylalanine	Proline	
Tryptophan	Serine	
Methionine		

Table 1. Essential, conditional and non-essential amino acids

©2022 ALLIANCE FOR NATURAL HEALTH INTERNATIONAL

Leave it to protein to do the heavy lifting

Proteins, or more specifically their sequences of amino acid chains, are responsible for so much more than building muscle. For a start, haemoglobin, necessary for transporting oxygen in the blood, is a protein. Almost all the complex biochemical reactions that take place in the body require enzymes to catalyse (make happen) the reaction and almost all enzymes are proteins. Protein not only provides fuel (energy) for our immune system, one of our most important defence enzymes, lysozyme, is a protein. Antibodies, necessary to protect us against infection, are also proteins.

Then there are signal/messenger proteins, like the hormones, insulin and secretin; lipoproteins in all our cell membranes and mucoproteins found in the synovial fluid that lubricates our joints. The proteins in our blood, albumin and globulin, maintain pressure and fluid/acid/alkaline balance as well as transporting ions, hormones and lipids (fats). Keratin, that maintains our skin, hair and nails is a protein, as are collagen and elastin. The latter being essential for forming strong white and yellow fibres in our tendons, cartilage, bone, ligaments and joint capsules.

If you're over 40 you may be uncomfortably reminded about the effects of collagen loss when you look in the mirror! If nothing else, it's a good motivation to keep your protein levels adequate and maintain good gut function, normal levels of stomach acid and steer clear of antacids (or PPIs). Without stomach acid (hydrochloric acid, HCl) you can't break the proteins down into their amino acid constituents and free them for use in the body, let alone the suite of other serious adverse effects that PPIs bring with them. In a bid to balance the equation, the market in collagen protein supplements is booming. Although any complete (containing all 9 essential amino acids) protein powder supplement will not only help keep your collagen strong and supple, it will also support all of the other functions that proteins perform in your body. Those with a really impaired gut may want to take an amino acid powder supplement so all the heavy lifting has been done already and they're then easier to absorb.

Structural proteins are involved in building muscles and tissues, with around 50% of the total body protein being muscle protein. This makes muscles effectively the body's long-term 'storage organ' for protein, leaving the amino acid pool as the short-term, easy access store. That's why when you're short on protein, your body will break down (catabolise) your muscle tissue to free proteins for other essential functions. Contractile proteins, such as actin and myosin, provide the ability for muscles to move. Proteins also play an integral role in the function of the cell in terms of of signalling and transport of small molecules through the cell wall.

These are just a few top line functions of protein to underpin that we would quite simply cease to exist without them.

How much is enough?

The World Health Organization (WHO) has set a minimum adult requirement for protein of 0.83 grams per kg of body weight (0.83 g/kg bw) per day. No need to memorise this term, but this calculation is based on a protein digestibility-corrected amino acid score value of 1.0, which means it's based on complete protein with both a high biological value (BV) and high digestibility eg. animal protein sources. It also applies to healthy adults, young ones at that, and not ones that are engaged in a lot of physical activity. The BV is a measure of the proportion of absorbed protein from a food which becomes incorporated into the proteins of the organism's body. The WHO's minimum level for protein for an adult also takes into account the digestibility of the protein source.

If you're vegetarian or vegan, you will need to increase the WHO's minimum level as plant proteins are often incomplete (don't contain the full group of essential amino acids), have reduced digestibility (eg. anti-nutrients: lectins, phytates, saponins and a lower BV, varying from around 0.60 to 0.75 (also sometimes expressed out of 100 as 60 to 75). That compares with 1.0 or 100 for egg white. It's also important to note that the WHO minimum is purely to maintain life without severe deficiency diseases like kwashiorkor or protein-energy malnutrition. The levels set by the WHO and other health authorities are certainly not about reaching and maintaining optimal or vibrant health from cradle to grave.

We can't ignore the importance of protein quality either, which includes its bioavailability once eaten. Bioavailability refers to the proportion of protein that can be absorbed from the diet and utilised in the body, taking into account digestibility, chemical integrity, and the lack of factors that can interfere with metabolism eg. food processing, non-nutritive additives, plant anti-nutrients and cooking methods (high temperatures denature and destroy proteins).

So, what should you aim for? Many practitioners use 1.0 g/kg bw per day for an adult as a minimum level of protein, but regularly recommend 1.2-1.4 g/kg bw for those with increased need. The highest figure being more common for physically active people, the elderly who have a reduced ability to absorb protein, or those with short-term, increased needs (illness, acute stress, wound healing etc). These levels are based on adults without kidney disease, but protein adequacy is also associated with age, level of health, gut function and individual requirement. Athletes will be on higher levels still because of their unique demand - up to 1.8 g/kg bw for power and strength athletes.

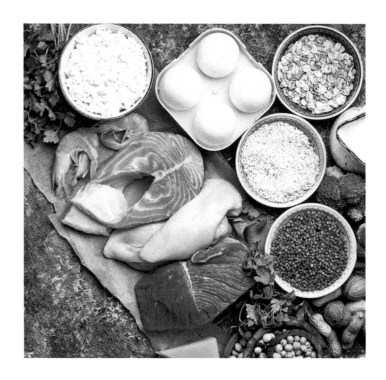

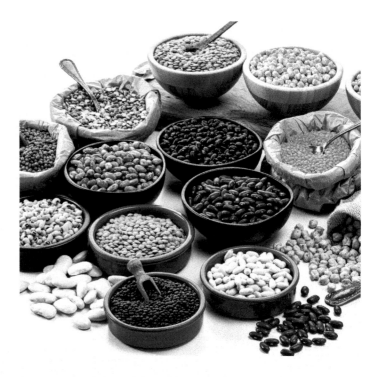

©2022 ALLIANCE FOR NATURAL HEALTH INTERNATIONAL

Amidst the many warnings about high protein levels causing kidney damage, it's worth remembering that 1.0 – 1.4 g/kg for a fit, active, adult is not high, and evidence shows that you don't need to be concerned if you have healthy kidneys. There is also plenty of evidence to show the benefits of having adequate protein in managing healthy blood glucose levels, reducing blood pressure and cardiovascular risk, which are some of the biggest killers of our time.

Does excess protein turn to sugar?

Gluconeogenesis is the term given to the method by which the body creates glucose from non-carbohydrate molecules if insufficient energy is available. It takes place in the liver and technically certain protein breakdown substrates (glucogenic amino acids, all excepting leucine and lysine) from protein metabolism could be used to produce glucose. However, given that protein is so important to survival, the body places it very high in the hierarchy of essential nutrients so you'd have to be eating a lot in the absence of any fats or carbs for this to happen. Putting cancer to one side, it

seems that warnings about protein being like another form of sugar are repeated frequently in a seeming attempt to admonish meat eaters or consumers of protein supplements. Interestingly, this particular 'misinformation' appears to date back to 1915, yet subsequent attempts to prove that protein intake influences blood glucose levels have all failed. Researchers tried again in 2013 and were unable to find an effect, concluding that the roles of dietary (and body) proteins in generating significant amounts of glucose to maintain blood glucose levels is questionable. In the absence of cancer, at normal dietary levels as discussed above, you can put any fears aside that your protein will metabolise into another form of glucose.

Protein prioritisation

The major deficiency diseases associated with protein are well documented and well known to anyone who's seen reports on malnutrition in developing countries. What's less well known are the health implications for not reaching an adequate protein level for your individual needs on an ongoing basis. Here are just two examples to ponder.

Mental health problems are now an issue globally. Whilst there is increasing acknowledgment from the mainstream about the potential role of the microbiome in depression, very little is being said about protein. Yet, the amino acid methionine helps the body produce SAMe (S-adenosyl-L-methionine) which has been shown to be as effective as antidepressants in alleviating depression. It's also been used in the treatment of psychiatric illnesses and is now being considered for Parkinson's disease. Methionine also supports immune function, detoxification and metabolism, which in the body's hierarchy of survival, trump feeling happy and balanced. So, a bit like looking in your bank account and seeing insufficient funds for all your bills, you're most likely going to prioritise paying the ones that could get you into real trouble and try and negotiate with the rest. The body does the same and most often, it's our emotional balance, mood and mental health that take a back seat because they're not likely to kill you.

Carnosine is a natural antioxidant that our body makes out of the amino acids, histidine and alanine. It's also an anti-glycation (AGEs) substance that's found in body tissues but primarily the brain and muscle cells (the heart too) and is important for muscle physiology as well as protecting us against age related diseases like heart disease, type 2 diabetes and Alzheimer's. But histidine is also involved with our immune response to allergens through its metabolism to the neurotransmitter histamine, as well as making stomach acid. Using the previous analogy, you might now start to see how we might make ourselves vulnerable through insufficient intake of protein. The body will always prioritise function according to its relevance to survival. It's worth mentioning that histidine is plentiful in most diets, but is often deficient in plant-based, especially vegan, diets. Therefore, supplementation with beta-alanine is considered especially important for vegan athletes.

Intuitive animals

Animals are so tuned into the need to find foods with adequate protein that it informs their foraging and alters food choice behaviours. Given that proteins have priority in the diet second only to energy, foods that yield the complete suite of essential amino acids must be found or animals (and humans!) start breaking down our own proteins. Scientists have found that the brains of animals are so attuned, that they can assess an amino acid deficient meal in 20 mins. Amazingly, within 2 hours their sensory cues are then associated with that food leading to a learned aversion for the future.

Would that we were so tuned in!

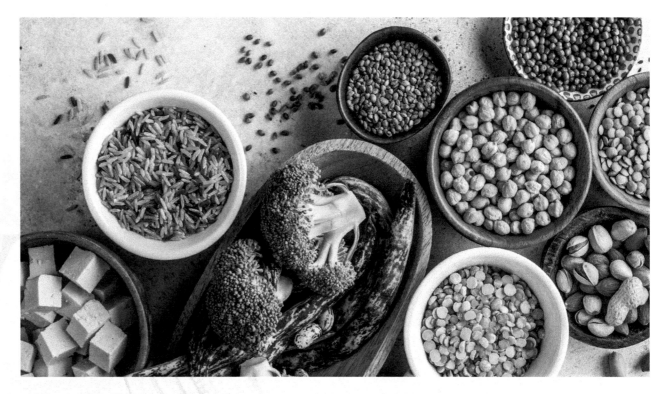

©2022 ALLIANCE FOR NATURAL HEALTH INTERNATIONAL

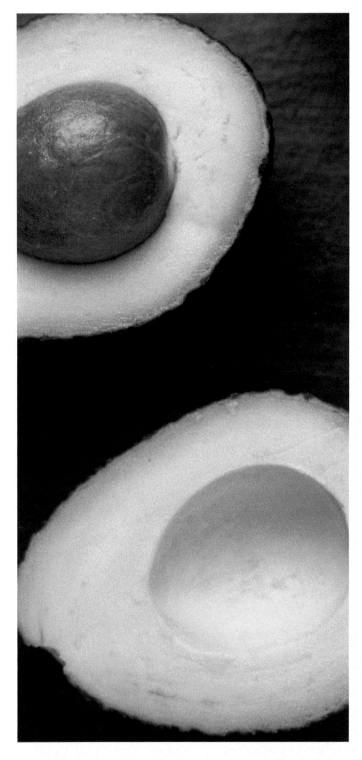

Macronutrients
2. Fats

Let's get something straight at the outset: eating fat — not even saturated fat — doesn't make you fat! That's despite what you may be reading in the media or being told by your dietitian. Fats have been touted as the bad boys on the nutritional block courtesy of some bad science in the 60's and 70's. Luckily, we now have much more accurate nutritional science to explain why you follow a fat-free diet at your peril. In fact, far from being foe, fats are friends, but just like you choose your friends carefully, so too with your dietary fats.

The skinny...

Fat is one of three essential macro nutrients along with protein and carbs. Apart from providing metabolic energy (fuel), fats play many important and active roles in the healthy functioning of our body. Most people believe fat is inert and that fat (adipose) tissue is just a storage place for excess calories. Whilst that's one function, it's only a small part of the role that fat plays in our health. What's more important to understand is that adipose tissue is actually a complex and metabolically dynamic endocrine organ in itself orchestrating multiple essential metabolic processes in the body. And the biggie - fat doesn't make you fat! It's carbs, and the sugars they yield, that deserve the blame.

Fuelling with the right fats

Despite what we're still told by governments and conventional dietetics, fat is not a dietary choice. It's an essential nutrient that's intimately entwined with our evolutionary history and our need for healthy fats today is largely unchanged.

Why? Because over millennia, our bodies have developed very intelligent systems for turning the food we eat into the energy we need to run all of our internal metabolism. Nature has evolved us in such a way to make fats our primary fuel for sustained energy. In our earlier history as hunter/gatherers before the development of agriculture around 12,000 years ago, we actually had very little in the way of simple sugars available to us. But we were very active, and our survival depended on us maintaining our energy levels over long periods - often in the absence of food. We did this through eating fats and burning fats, not carbs, for fuel.

Some healthy fats that deserve hero status in your diet:

THE MUFAS (monounsaturated fats)	Olive oil
	Peanut oil (if not allergic)
	Sesame oil (sparingly)
	Avocados
	Olives
	Nuts (almonds, peanuts, macadamia nuts, hazelnuts, pecans) (if not allergic)
	Nut butters (if not allergic)
THE PUFAS (polyunsaturated fats)	Walnuts
	Flaxseed
	Fatty fish (salmon, tuna, mackerel, herring, trout, sardines)
THE SAFAS (saturated fats)	High-fat cuts of marbled meat (beef, lamb, pork) - with the fat inside the meat, not all around the outside
	Chicken with the skin on
	Whole-fat dairy products (milk and cream) - if you're not intolerant
	Butter
	Cheese
	Coconut oil
	Lard

©2022 ALLIANCE FOR NATURAL HEALTH INTERNATIONAL

Different shades of fat

Let's have a look at the fat in our body before we go much further. For some time we thought there were two main types, white and brown, but now you can add beige fat to the list. Each has its own unique function:

- White fat is the most prevalent in the body - think of the fat under the skin that you can pinch (or grab!). Far from being inert storage, white fat's functions include the secretion of hormones, growth factors, enzymes, cytokines (immune system messengers) as well as physically protecting organs, energy storage and indirectly, temperature regulation

- Brown fat is 'active' fat found primarily in the front and back of the neck and upper back. Babies and children have higher levels of brown fat, which decreases significantly as you age or if you're sedentary. Its main purpose is to regulate body temperature by burning calories to generate heat and keep us warm without shivering. We now know that we can stimulate brown fat production in adults by using cold therapy like ice baths, ice challenges and cold water showers. The latter made more effective by allowing yourself to air dry!

- Beige fat is a type of adipose tissue found embedded in white fat. It's a relatively new discovery and research indicates that it's also involved in temperature regulation, albeit differently to brown fat. You can also encourage more beige fat cells by exposing yourself to cold, aka the Wim Hof method.

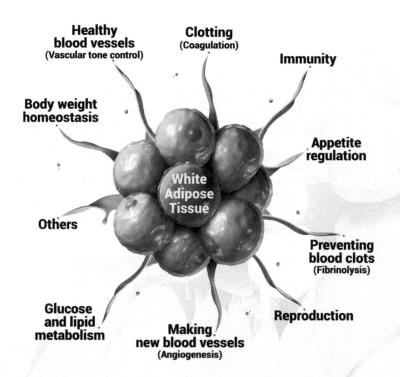

Figure 2. Physiological functions of white adipose tissue (WAT)

Location, location, location

Where fat is located in our body makes a huge difference in how it impacts our health. Subcutaneous fat (WAT) is located under the skin (can you pinch an inch or more?), whereas visceral fat (VAT) is found inside our abdominal cavity wrapping around and crowding out our internal organs. Too much tummy fat being the most dangerous kind carrying the highest risk of future health problems.

Visceral fat is often described as 'angry' fat because it pumps out inflammatory chemical messengers that incites the body to dysfunction. Imagine a large group of people shoved in a tiny space. Instead of increasing the space or reducing the number of people, you add more people. They're going to get angry and start shouting about their experience, which then sets off the people in the nearby spaces - bad news travels fast - inciting a chain reaction of not so nice effects. Like an angry mob on the rampage in your body. This is pretty much what happens when your fat cells are forced to grow, and grow, in the tight space of the abdomen. VAT is very active fat sending out a cascade of inflammatory signals that the immune system has to act upon. However, the good news is that VAT is extremely receptive to diet and lifestyle changes, particularly if you can include some moderate endurance activity like walking or cycling that lasts longer than 90 mins once or twice a week.

Brown and beige 'thermogenic' fat can be stimulated and maintained by being active and not being afraid of the cold eg. ice baths.

A chemical factory

Healthy adipose tissue has many benefits and secretes a range of bioactive substances:

- Leptin - is a peptide (from protein), but it functions like a hormone. It's often called the 'satiety hormone' because it regulates the size of the fat deposits in the body. Leptin is part of our evolutionary survival response and can regulate energy intake and fat stores within a narrow margin. When fat mass decreases, the level of leptin decreases and the appetite is stimulated until fat is regained. There is also a decrease in body temperature and energy expenditure is reduced.

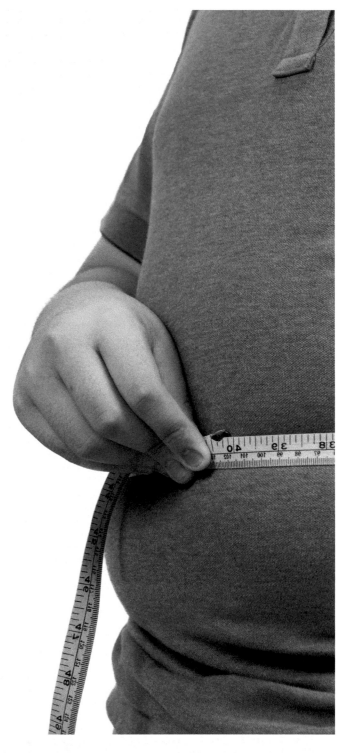

©2022 ALLIANCE FOR NATURAL HEALTH INTERNATIONAL

- When fat deposits increase, so do leptin levels, suppressing appetite until weight loss occurs. Interestingly, leptin also plays a role in puberty as a woman requires sufficient fat stores if she's to nourish a foetus and ensure the survival of the human race. When leptin levels are persistently high from overeating, the leptin receptors become 'deaf' resulting in reduced sensitivity to the hormone — a condition we refer to as leptin resistence. The absence of leptin, or fully functioning leptin receptors, can lead to uncontrolled eating, which in turn increases the risk of obesity.

- Adiponectin – like leptin, is also secreted by fat cells. It plays a role in the regulation of blood glucose and helps burn fat for energy. Low levels of adiponectin have been implicated in the development of obesity and insulin resistance.

Carrying excessive amounts of VAT and WAT, increases the production and secretion of inflammatory 'messengers' like cytokines (eg, tumour necrosis factor-α, interleukin-6, leptin, nuclear factor kappa beta) as well as hormones and other signalling molecules as detailed below. The result of this disturbed signalling causes metabolic havoc leading to a rash of chronic diseases eg. obesity, type 2 diabetes, heart disease, Alzheimer's, dementia, osteoporosis and hormonal imbalance.

Low fat - a huge public health mistake

Low fat public health policies followed by most governments around the world from the 1970s are beginning to look like one of the biggest mistakes in the history of public health.

The decision to demonise fats and link them to heart disease was borne out of a kind of join-the-dots approach to science. Believe it or not, public health authorities and world class scientists managed to add 2 and 2 and get 5. They bought in heavily to Dr Ancel Key's misrepresented Seven Countries study and the cholesterol hypothesis for heart disease. Fats, and saturated fats in particular, were made public enemy number 1

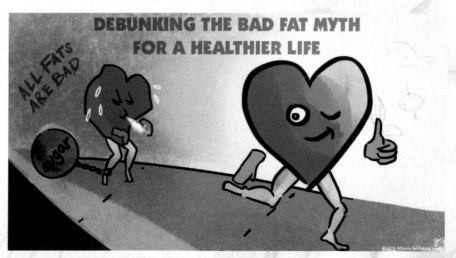

because intake was wrongly related to cholesterol levels in our body. The 'cholesterol-heart disease' hypothesis quietly morphed into the 'saturated fat-heart disease' hypothesis. Then, without any reliable scientific facts to support either, saturated fat in the diet and high cholesterol in the body became the primary scapegoats for dealing with the biggest killer disease in the industrialised world.

It worked a treat if you happened to be selling a cholesterol-lowering drug like a statin. And, perversely, few thought it was odd that statins weren't solving the heart disease epidemic despite them being dished out like Smarties. Anyway, the cat is out of the bag now, and while there hasn't been any formal acknowledgement of wrongdoing from the scientific community and governments involved, fats and saturated fats are not being maligned quite in the way they were. But in most parts of the world, there's still a long way to go.

Luckily, the nutritional science community has established that the fatty acid profile that we consume is key. Like with proteins, it's not just about the quantity, the quality is equally, if not more, important. This involves consuming the right amounts of monounsaturated, polyunsaturated and saturated fats. When societies went low fat (and unfortunately too many still consider low-fat foods as healthy options), the two things we did were switch to highly processed vegetable oils, margarines and spreads rich in Omega-6 fatty acids and increase our consumption of sugars and highly processed grains.

As we've already discussed, the energy from fats is over double that from carbs and protein. Pull saturated fats out of the diet and you've got to replace this energy gap with something. The big food companies have managed to exploit what's called the 'bliss point' for all its worth, finding that special combination of sugar, salt and fats (polyunsaturated, highly processed vegetables ones that were then considered healthy) that makes it really hard for most people to flick the off switch and stop eating.

Most western societies have massively ramped up the amount of processed foods and reduced the amount made at home. Many have also become a whole lot more sedentary. Looking back, we can now see that increasing refined carbs in a sedentary, overweight population does a whole lot more metabolic damage than higher saturated fat in a more active, normal weight one. The result has been that our waistlines have continued growing and our metabolism has become so imbalanced that our hormones have lost the ability to regulate appetite or energy storage and usage efficiently. You can see the effect that this has had when you look at the rising levels of chronic disease.

©2022 ALLIANCE FOR NATURAL HEALTH INTERNATIONAL

Macronutrients
3. Carbohydrates

We're often told that carbs are an essential food group, necessary for energy metabolism, health and wellbeing. Moreover, mainstream dietitians would have you believe that a large part of your daily diet should be made up of carbohydrates. But is this right? And will you suffer or thrive by cutting out – or down on – carbs?

The low-down on carbs

Carbohydrates are biomolecules made up of carbon, hydrogen and oxygen. Put simply they are a form of stored energy packaged especially into plants. Today, the term carbohydrate is generally used to refer to starchy foods such as grain-based bread, pasta and cereals; root vegetables like potatoes, carrots, parsnips and beetroot; and sugars. However, all vegetables are sources of complex carbs, so even when you cut out starchy carbs, you're never carb-free, unless you also cut out all vegetables, fruit, mushrooms, algae (eg. seaweeds), herbs and spices. When we eat plants, we eat carbs, even though people don't seem to think of vegetables as being sources of carbohydrate. But, because food is information, different types of carbs, along with other components in those foods or associated meals, speak a different language in the body.

The simplest form of carbohydrates are single unit sugars known as monosaccharides. These link together to form complex carbohydrates known as disaccharides, oligosaccharides (also known as prebiotics as they provide food for our gut microbiota) and polysaccharides, which can be further categorised into starch and non-starch polysaccharides. The time it takes for your digestive system to break down carbohydrate units into useable glucose is dependent on how simple or complex it is (ie. the length or branching of the carbon backbone). The more complex the chain, the longer it takes to breakdown and enter your bloodstream, hence, the more stable your blood sugar. The resulting glucose is then absorbed into your bloodstream ready to be used by your cells to make energy in the form of adenosine triphosphate (ATP). ATP, as we've outlined, is our body's energy currency, used to fuel the myriad functional and metabolic processes that allow us to perform optimally in dynamic (ever changing) environments.

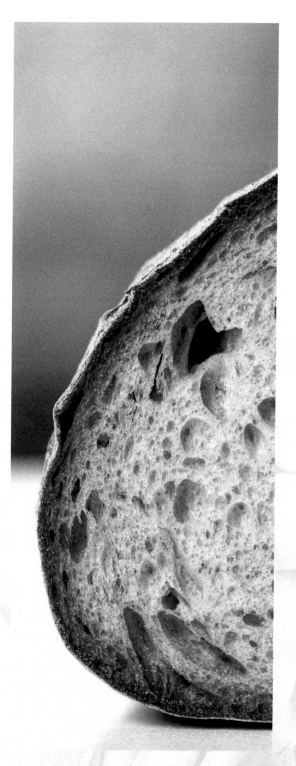

It's important to remember that whilst plant foods are carbohydrate dominant, they generally also contain varying levels of protein and fats. It's the combination of macronutrients (carbs, proteins and fats) in a food source (or meal) that influences the rate at which they are broken down and therefore its effect on our blood glucose levels.

Many carbs in plant foods are undigestible for us, but are necessary to feed our gut microbiome. Most oligosaccharides (except maltodextrin), some starches and all non-starch polysaccharides are resistant to digestion. They pass into the large bowel where they are fermented by our gut bugs to make short-chain fatty acids (SCFAs) providing energy both for us and the variety of organisms in our gut. These resistant carbs also provide essential fibre which promotes healthy detoxification and elimination.

Delivering essential phytonutrients, compounds that help protect against disease and promote health, plants are integral to good health. They are nature's pharmacy – our first medicine, so it's no surprise that the non-nutritive, medicinal consumption of a diverse range of plant foods has been long known in our nearest non-human primate relatives,

CLASS	EXAMPLE	DESCRIPTION	
Monosaccharides	Glucose, fructose, galactose	Single unit sugars	Digestible
Disaccharides	Sucrose, lactose, maltose	Double unit sugars	Digestible
Oligosaccharides	Fructo-oligosaccharides, inulin, maltodextrins, raffinose, verbascose, stachyose	3-9 sugar unit (monosaccharide) chains	Indigestible (fermented in gut)
Starch polysaccharides	Amylose, amylopectin, maltodextrins	10 or more sugar unit (monosaccharide) chains	Indigestible (fermented in gut)
Non-starch polysaccharides (dietary fibre)	Cellulose, pectins, hemicelluloses, gums, inulin	Dietary fibre. Humans cannot digest, but various gut bacteria can	Indigestible (fermented in gut)

Table 2. Classes and digestibility of carbohydrates

chimpanzees, bonobos and gorillas. Whilst we benefit hugely from leafy and coloured vegetables, the vast majority of us can get along very nicely without the starchy carbs that come from grains and large amounts of root vegetables. Recreating our 'diet of origin' with the Food4Health Guide and becoming metabolically flexible, where the burning of fat yields ketones as an additional source of ATP, with glucose from carbs as a secondary source, helps promote long-term health, build muscle and reduce the effects of ageing.

©2022 ALLIANCE FOR NATURAL HEALTH INTERNATIONAL

Carbohydrate loading

Talking of fuel, in energy terms 1 gram of carbohydrate or protein provides 4 kcal, whereas 1 gram of fat provides us with 9 kcal, making fats a far more efficient energy source. It's no wonder that burning fat for energy was our evolutionary norm and the choice for survival.

You may have seen the terms 'glycaemic index' and 'glycaemic load' attributed to foods that are high in carbs. Carb-containing foods are also described as being high or low glycaemic. The Glycaemic Index (GI) is a way of ranking foods according to how quickly they increase blood glucose levels. Foods with a GI of less than 55 are digested, absorbed and metabolised more slowly causing a slower increase in blood glucose and therefore insulin levels. An extension of this is glycaemic load (GL), which considers the quantity and quality of carbs eaten giving a more accurate picture of how high your blood sugar levels go and for how long after eating a typical serving of that food. The rate that your blood sugar level rises and for how long is called the 'glycaemic response'. A disordered and dysfunctional glycaemic response that's allowed to continue for years is central to the creation of diseases like obesity, type 2 diabetes, cardiovascular disease and even many cancers.

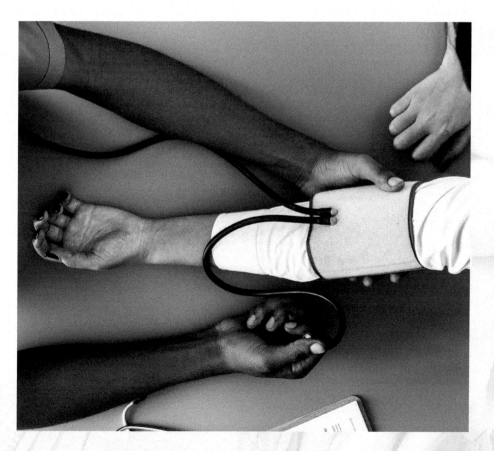

FOOD	GI (AVERAGE)	SERVE SIZE (G)	AVAILABLE CARBOHYDRATE	GL (PER SERVING)
GRAINS/STARCHES				
Rice noodles	61	180	39	23
Spaghetti, white	44	180	48	21
Cornflakes	81	30	26	21
Boiled white rice	64	150	38	20
Baked potato	60	150	30	18
Instant porridge	66	250	26	17
Muesli	66	30	24	17
Corn chips	63	50	26	17
Sweet potato	61	150	28	17
Boiled white potatoes	50	150	28	14
Wheat biscuits (aka Weetabix)	70	30	19	13
Porridge, whole oats	58	250	22	13
White bread toasted	73	30	15	11
White bread	73	30	14	10
Popcorn	72	20	11	10
Wholewheat bread	71	30	13	9
Sourdough rye bread	53	30	12	6
BAKED GOODS				
Doughnut	76	47	23	17
Sponge cake	46	63	36	17
Croissant	67	57	26	17
Blueberry muffin	59	57	29	17

©2022 ALLIANCE FOR NATURAL HEALTH INTERNATIONAL

FOOD	GI (AVERAGE)	SERVE SIZE (G)	AVAILABLE CARBOHYDRATE	GL (PER SERVING)
SUGARS				
Honey	55	25	18	10
Sucrose	68	10	10	7
Fructose	19	10	10	2
Agave nectar	11	10	8	1
CHOCOLATE				
Milk chocolate (Cadbury's)	49	50	30	14
Plain chocolate	34	50	22	7
FRUIT				
Orange juice	50	250	26	13
Banana	52	120	24	12
Apple juice	40	250	29	12
Pineapple, raw	59	120	13	7
Apple	38	120	15	6
Kiwi	79	120	12	6
Orange	42	120	11	5
Watermelon	72	120	6	4
Pear	33	120	13	4
Cherries	22	120	12	3

FOOD	GI (AVERAGE)	SERVE SIZE (G)	AVAILABLE CARBOHYDRATE	GL (PER SERVING)
VEGETABLES				
Parsnips	97	80	12	12
Sweetcorn	54	80	17	9
Chickpeas	28	150	30	8
Lentils	29	150	18	5
Cooked carrots	47	80	6	3
Green peas	48	80	7	3
DAIRY (INC PLANT 'MILK')				
Ice-cream	61	50	13	8
Soy milk	36	250	18	6
Skimmed milk	32	250	13	4
Yogurt	36	200	9	3
Full fat milk	27	250	12	3
NUTS				
Cashew Nuts (salted)	22	50	13	3
Peanuts	23	50	6	1

 ©2022 ALLIANCE FOR NATURAL HEALTH INTERNATIONAL

Not all carbs speak the same 'language'

The kicker in all of this is it's not just how we process carbs internally, but also externally that makes the difference. Governments and mainstream dietitians would have you eating around 60% of your daily calories from carbs, and much of that from starchy carbs in the form of wholegrains. Yet it's these kinds of foods, wholegrain or not, that we're encouraged to eat that create a high glycaemic load (GL).

Regular consumption of high GI and GL foods that are also highly processed creates such frequent blood sugar elevation that the pancreas has to work overtime to make enough insulin to bring the blood sugar levels down. The over-exposure to insulin then starts to make cells under-responsive to insulin's blood sugar lowering effects so more is produced - and 'insulin resistance', the precursor to type 2 diabetes, develops. The resulting elevated levels of insulin tell the body to store fat, so it becomes ever harder to mobilise fats and burn them for fuel.

How does this all feel? Well, the yo-yoing of blood sugar levels contributes to tiredness, lack of concentration and more sugar cravings. Appetite regulation goes haywire, so you no longer feel full even when you've just eaten and have ample energy on-board. You think by grabbing that quick carb fix, be it a chocolate bar or other high glycaemic fix, you'll feel better. You do - for a short while - but when your blood sugar crashes an hour or so later, you do it all over again. The cycle goes on - until you make yourself properly ill, with type 2 diabetes and/or obesity, and a psychological craving for sweet, sugary, refined carb 'comfort foods'.

A perfect example of the kind of food that feeds into this pattern of eating is the so-called 'healthy' breakfast cereal, so highly processed you may as well eat a bowl of sugar as far as your body is concerned. Contrast that with minimally processed wholefood sources of carbs like steel cut oats and a handful of berries and it's an entirely different kettle of fish as far as your blood sugar response is concerned.

The infiltration of our diet by Big Food's processed and ultra-processed, calorific, nutrient-deficient carbs is driving the obesity crisis and in turn insulin resistance, Metabolic Syndrome (pre-diabetes),

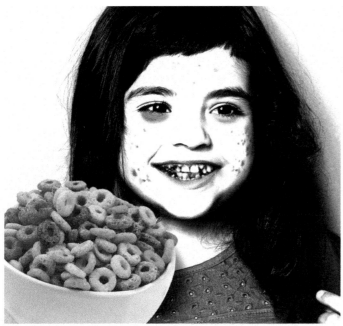

Adulterated Poison.

Top ingredient by weight = sugar. This breakfast 'delight' is then laced with highly processed carbs . Even if the pack claims there's "wholegrain" inside, the ultra-processing will spike your kids blood sugar just like sugar. **Call that a double whammy!** Just what a child doesn't need midmorning as the insulin spike crashes the blood sugar level to the point where your kids need to function at school drives him or her to devour another refined carb in the perfectly timed midmorning break.

If that wasn't enough, these coloured loops also deliver partially hydrogenated and trans fats, as well as a trio of artificial colours that have been related to increased cancer risk or **Attention Deficit Hyperactivity Disorder (ADHD).**

All of this amounts to a child's worse possible breakfast - to which he or she can become addicted. Don't be taken in by 'wholegrain' or 'high fibre' - this stuff is pure, adulterated, addictive poison for kids.

KEEP OUT OF REACH OF CHILDREN!

A public service announcement from the Alliance for Natural Health International

type 2 diabetes and a swathe of other chronic diseases. Despite continued insistence by health authorities that the driver of cardiovascular disease is saturated fat, recent research shows the real culprit is elevated blood sugars and insulin coming from over-dependence on starchy, refined, processed carbs.

In addition, the type of carbohydrate we eat has a huge influence on the health of our gut microbiota. Diets high in ultra-processed carbs affect the microbial composition of our guts. This impacts our immune system and damages the delicate lining of our gut, leaving us at higher risk of developing an increasing range of autoimmune diseases. We need to remember that when we eat, we dine with trillions of microbes that require certain foods to keep them healthy. If they're healthy, they keep us healthy. It's meant to be win-win.

Is your brain really screaming for sugar?

Our brain is the organ that requires more energy than any other in the body. Outdated dietetic science would have us believe its preferred fuel is glucose, but if this were the case, the human race wouldn't be here today. Our evolutionary adaptations enable us to work just as well, if not better, on a blend of ketones and minimal amounts of glucose. Burning fat to make ketones is far cleaner, creating much less oxidative damage in the body than burning sugars, which can lead to the accumulation of advanced glycation end products (AGEs) promoting chronic disease.

The controversy around low carb diets continues to rage. Not least, in part because there is no clear, universally accepted definition of what is meant by a 'low carb diet' or a 'low carb high fat' (LCHF) diet with recommendations ranging from less than 40% to less than 5% by energy (kcal or kJ). The Food4Health guidelines recommend 25% by energy, recognising the importance of fibre from vegetables and fruit on our gut health - that's less than half the amount recommended by most governments.

Is it in your genes?

Whilst it's true to say that while your genes may load the gun, it's your diet, lifestyle and environment that pulls the trigger. Advances in nutrigenomics means that we can now screen people to look for those that are genetically vulnerable to becoming overweight because they are predisposed to being more intolerant to carbs than others.

A sensitivity to carbs, sometimes referred to as 'carbotoxicity' in the scientific literature, is an important reason why some people really struggle to be healthy eating vegan or even vegetarian, despite a deep desire to give up eating animal produce. The vast majority of plant-based protein foods, with a few exceptions, come with a hefty helping of carbohydrates. Often, eating a vegan diet that contains no animal products can be low in protein and fat and high in carbs. This configuration of macronutrients can trigger some people into metabolic dysregulation and, over time, into a place of increased systemic (internal, whole body) inflammation. For these people, it can become hard to keep the fire of inflammation inside their bodies at bay and maintain

©2022 ALLIANCE FOR NATURAL HEALTH INTERNATIONAL

a healthy weight with good lean muscle tone. This is one reason why the most committed vegans may end up going back to eating some animal protein after a number of years – and then get their health back. However, for those who choose to remain 100% plant based it can be helpful to keep levels of allergens and anti-nutrients as low as possible. In particular, this means avoiding gluten (in gluten-containing grains) and using a pressure cooker to neutralise anti-nutrients like lectins in pulses and beans. These two steps can go a long way to helping to support gut health and reduce the risk of intestinal permeability ('leaky gut') – both of which are big drivers of systemic inflammation.

If you're a vegan or vegetarian who wants to 'go keto', it's wholly possible to be fully plant-based and low carb. It just takes a bit more work to make sure your meals are balanced, colourful and not too carb-heavy, especially avoiding refined and starchy carbs. Eating the Food4Health way gives your body lots of non-starchy, above-ground veg along with a bit of fruit. This provides the perfect, grain-free source of carbs for most people, also giving you lots of digestible and indigestible fibre that keeps your

gut and gut bacteria happy. Eating this way equips your body with all the nutrients and information it needs to optimise function and be well. It also gives you sufficient healthy fats to drive your fat-burning (beta oxidation), ketone-generating pathways. For vegetarians, eggs and dairy (if tolerated) can be very useful additions on the journey to keto-adaptation.

As our gene expression is driven by what we eat, how we move and behave and what we experience in life, it's very much within our control to create a different outcome. That includes making different choices about what, when and how we eat; when and how we move; when and how we respond to and recover from stress and how we limit our environmental toxin burden. This is good news and these tests should be more widely available. It's the future of personalised, individualised medicine. Health creation rather than disease management.

Are you carb intolerant?

The carb kings in most people's minds are grains and cereals with fruits and vegetables being overlooked. The interesting thing is that we have to start thinking a bit more about carbs because carbohydrate intolerance is a big issue in our modern world. In fact, we go so far as to say that carbohydrate intolerance is the single biggest driver of the obesity and type 2 diabetes epidemic that's sweeping the world.

This brief questionnaire won't take the place of genetic or functional testing, but it will give you an indication of dysfunction in how you process starchy or refined carbs. If you answer yes to any of these questions, it's likely you'll benefit from eating according to the Food4Health guide, but also from a 2-week exclusion of all grains, refined and starchy carbs.

Q1	Are you overweight or obese?
Q2	Has your doctor tested your haemoglobin A1c (HbA1c) levels lately? This gives information about your average blood sugar levels over the last 3 months. Was your level higher than 5.5 (with or without many sugary foods in your diet)?
Q3	Do you suffer from tiredness all the time?
Q4	Do you feel your energy saps away after eating a starchy-carb heavy meal?
Q5	Do you have cravings for sweets or starchy foods like bread and pasta?
Q6	Do you feel hungry soon after eating starchy or sugary foods e.g. pizza, pasta, sandwiches, cakes, biscuits?
Q7	Do you feel shaky, lightheaded or dizzy when you get hungry?
Q8	Do you feel 'hangry' when leaving gaps of more than 3 hours between eating?
Q9	Are you sedentary or exercise infrequently?
Q10	Do you suffer with brain fog, lack of concentration, depression, hormonal imbalance, aching or sleep problems?

Going 'cold turkey' for 14 days by cutting out grains, sugar (and all sugary foods), legumes (e.g. kidney beans, chickpeas, lentils etc), root vegetables (e.g. potatoes, carrots, parsnips, beetroot etc) and fruit and taking the questionnaire again, is an inexpensive way to determine if your relationship with carbs is healthy or toxic. You can also search for a functional medicine practitioner near you to help you through the process.

 ©2022 ALLIANCE FOR NATURAL HEALTH INTERNATIONAL

Changing the type and amount of carbohydrate foods in your diet, the way you prepare them and how often you eat them can be the difference between disease promotion and disease prevention.

Micronutrients

Nutritional science is helping us to realise that food is fundamentally a form of information for the body. A single, healthy meal with a bountiful supply of plant foods may contain many thousands of discrete naturally-occurring compounds that do a lot more than just provide energy to fuel the body. As you can see, the three main macronutrient groups, carbohydrates, fats and proteins, can all be used as energy sources. But the micronutrients, that may include essential fatty acids, plant (phyto-) nutrients, various fibres, enzymes, amino acids and other compounds, are needed to keep our bodies — despite changing environments and different forms of stress — in a balanced state (homeostasis). That's not only through the effect they have on our own cells, but also in how they affect the microbes in our gut that outnumber human cells 10 to 1.

Many of these bioactive compounds in our food act as signalling compounds that help regulate metabolic pathways. Very importantly, the quality of our diet affects the way in which our genes are expressed through epigenetic processes such as DNA methylation and histone modification that turn on or off particular genes, or for that matter, make some whisper or shout loudly. It is of course not our genes themselves that control our destiny, but the ways in which they are expressed. Interestingly, these modifications can also be transmitted to subsequent generations (at least 3 or 4). The rapidly emerging discipline of epigenetics reinforces diet and lifestyle based medicine as probably the most relevant form of medicine today, especially when our greatest health burdens relate to chronic, degenerative diseases like cancer, heart disease, type 2 diabetes and obesity, that are so often triggered by long-term patterns of poor diet and lifestyle choices.

Micronutrients are usually expressed in terms of essentiality. Essential nutrients are those you can't make in your body that are responsible for acute deficiency diseases like beri beri, scurvy or kwashiorkor disease. Non-essential

---

DO WE GET ALL WE NEED FROM OUR DIETS?

MACRONUTRIENTS
(grams of each per day)

- Protein
- (Water)
- Fats
- Carbohydrates

MICRONUTRIENTS
(milligrams or micrograms of each per day)

- Vitamins
- Phospholipids
- Minerals
- Enzymes
- Amino acids
- Microorganisms
- Fatty acids
- Nucleotides
- Fibres
- Cofactors
- Phytochemicals

MICRONUTRIENTS OUR BODIES NEED

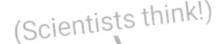

(Scientists think!)

ESSENTIAL NUTRIENTS	CONDITIONALLY (SEMI) ESSENTIAL NUTRIENTS	NON-ESSENTIAL NUTRIENTS
Must be consumed in food throughout life	Must be consumed in food stages at some stages of life	Not required for short-term survival
Insufficiency may lead to serious deficiency diseases	Insufficiency may lead to health deficits or chronic disease(s)	Insufficiency may lead to health deficits, chronic or degenerative disease(s), especially in later life

ESSENTIAL NUTRIENTS

Examples

14 vitamins
20+ minerals
9 amino acids
phenylalanine, valine, tryptophan, methionine, leucine, isoleucine, lysine and histidine
Essential fatty acids (EFAs)
alpha-linolenic acid (ALA), linoleic acid (LA)

CONDITIONALLY (SEMI) ESSENTIAL NUTRIENTS

Examples

6 amino acids
arginine, cysteine, glycine, glutamine, proline, tyrosine
Nucleotides
Omega-3 fatty acids
docosahexaenoic acid (DHA), eicosapentaenoic acid (EPA)

NON-ESSENTIAL NUTRIENTS

Examples

5 amino acids
alanine, aspartic acid, asparagine, glutamic acid, serine
Thousands of bioactive compounds in botanicals
phytonutrients
Polysaccharides
Bacteria
Fungi
Microalgae
Enzymes
Glandular extracts

©2022 ALLIANCE FOR NATURAL HEALTH INTERNATIONAL

and conditionally-essential micronutrients are often overlooked by conventional health care, but deficiencies of these nutrients give rise to the massive burden of chronic disease. Our Food4Health guidelines are designed to help you avoid deficiencies in any category. But where you may need more, given the declining soil quality, industrial agricultural practices and increasing demands of modern life, then you will see that dietary supplements are catered for alongside herbs and spices in the segment devoted to concentrated sources of nutrients.

Put simply, and as a general rule of thumb, the more diverse the range of foods that we eat and the greater the range of nutrients, the more protection our body has against disease — and the better its ability to promote wellness.

Miracle gifts from plants

Phytochemicals is the term used to describe plant-based nutrients. They remind us that not all chemicals are dangerous! These are the compounds that give fruits and vegetables their colour, flavour (including bitterness) and smell. In the plant, these phytochemicals defend against disease, attack by insects and microbes, as well as environmental stressors such as ultra-violet light, cold, heat, lack of water, poor soil quality and pollution.

Different plants have developed specific phytonutrients for particular defensive needs eg. resveratrol in grapes and berries to protect against fungal infection, stress and UV light. In us, these phytochemicals provide essential protection against diseases eg. cancer, neurodegeneration,

diabetes and cardiovascular disease to name a few. The more we reduce the diversity of foods we eat, breed plants and raise animals to increase corporate profits, pander to our sweet tooth and declining palates with sweeter fruits and vegetables, highly processed foods and high-yield crops — the more we remove the very nutrients our body has evolved with to keep it healthy and disease-free.

Eat a rainbow every day

Diversity and quality are key to making any dietary plan really work for you. The wider the range of foods we eat, the more nutrients we get and the more protection we have against developing chronic disease. The Food4Health Guide is heavily plant based because by eating a broad range of plant foods, we benefit from a whole matrix of different nutrients.

Did you know that your body and its internal and external environment is actually an entire and complete ecosystem? You have an entire world within you – and that world is heavily dependent on what you eat. Your world consists of you and more than a trillion microbes that live within and on you. Without microbes, we'd simply cease to exist, such is our close relationship. Plant foods are so much more than fuel or energy for the body – they are information. This is why we make plants the foundation of our Food4Health Guide as eating this way is so consistently linked to long-term health and wellbeing.

What our personal ecosystems really need to achieve balance is the information contained in a diverse range of coloured plant foods on a daily basis – a whole 'rainbow' of vegetables and fruits. Making sure you have sufficient fresh, plant foods for fermentable fibres in your diet is the first step to cultivating a healthy gut microbiome too.

The 6 colours of nature's palette are red, orange, yellow, green, white/tan/brown and blue/purple/black. They're out there in the range of fruits and vegetables available to us, and each colour delivers particular plant compounds (phytonutrients) that have specific functions in the body, promoting health and protecting against disease.

Our DNA is encoded to respond positively to colourful foods. If we've been introduced to these foods from early childhood then we tend to find eating diverse, 'rainbow' coloured diets more appealing. They assure us that the food is ripe, ready to eat and healthful, plus they stimulate our appetite. Think about the succulence of a fresh sun-ripened orange or nectarine, the lushness of a bundle of green, leafy watercress or the regal purple of blueberries fresh from the bush.

Nutrition research now tells us that it should be '6 colours every day' rather than the '5 A DAY' we keep hearing in the public health narrative. These are foods that have nourished us, healed us and ensured our survival through the ages.

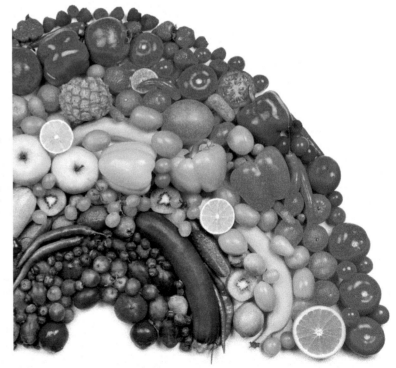

©2022 ALLIANCE FOR NATURAL HEALTH INTERNATIONAL

EAT A RAINBOW EVERY DAY

Consume foods which represent all 6 colour groups of the 'phytonutrient spectrum' each and every day!

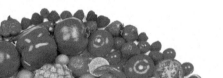

We would like to acknowledge the Institute for Functional Medicine (www.functionalmedicine.org) as the primary source of the information on the 'phytonutrient spectrum'.

RED FOODS

Beans (adzuki, kidney, red), Beetroot, Red peppers, Blood oranges, Cranberries, Cherries, Goji berries, Grapefruit (pink), Red apples, Red grapes, Red onions, Red plums, Pomegranate, Potatoes (red skin), Radicchio, Red cabbage, Red leaf lettuce, Radishes, Raspberries, Strawberries, Sweet red peppers, Rhubarb, Rooibos tea, Tomato, Watermelon

BENEFITS

Cancer protective, healthy inflammatory response, cell protection, gastrointestinal health, heart health, hormone balance, liver health

ORANGE FOODS

Apricots, Bell peppers (orange), Carrots, Grapefruit, Mango, Nectarine, Orange, Papaya, Pumpkin, Squash (Butternut/Acorn/Winter), Sweet Potato, Tangerines, Turmeric Root, Yams

BENEFITS

Cancer protective, immune health, cell protection, reduced all-cause mortality, immune health, reproductive health, skin health, source of pro-vitamin A

YELLOW FOODS

Apple, Banana, Bell peppers (yellow), Sweetcorn, Corn-on-the-cob, Chickpeas, Ginger root, Lemon, Millet, Pineapple, Popcorn

BENEFITS

Cancer protective, healthy inflammatory response, cell protection, cognition, skin health, eye health, heart/vascular health

GREEN FOODS

Apples (green), Artichoke, Asparagus, Avocado, Bamboo shoots, Bean sprouts, Bok Choy, Broccoli, Brussels sprouts, Cabbage (beet leaves, chard, dandelion leaves, kale, lettuce, mustard leaves, spinach, rocket, etc.), Celery, Cucumbers, Edemame (soybeans), Beans, Peas (e.g. green, mangetout), Green Tea, Lettuce, Limes, Okra, Olives (green), Rosemary, Spinach, Watercress

BENEFITS

Healthy inflammatory response, brain health, cell protection, skin health, hormone balance, heart health, liver health

WHITE/TAN/BROWN FOODS

Apples, Beans (butter, cannellini, etc), Cauliflower, Cinnamon, Clove, Coconut, Cocoa, Coffee, Dark Chocolate, Flaxseed, Garlic, Ginger, Hummus, Legumes (chickpeas, dried beans, Hummus, Houmous, lentils, Peanuts, etc), Mushrooms, Nuts (almonds, cashews, macadamias, pecans, walnuts), Onions, Pears, Seeds (flax, hemp, pumpkin, sesame, sunflower, etc), Shallots, Tahini, Tea (black, white), Whole Grains (amaranth, buckwheat, corn, millet, montina, oats, quinoa, rice, sorghum, teff – all naturally free of gluten)

BENEFITS

Cancer protective, anti-microbial, cell protection, gastrointestinal health, heart health, liver health, hormone balance

BLUE/PURPLE/BLACK FOODS

Aubergine, Berries (blue/black), Cabbage (purple), Carrots (purple), Cauliflower (purple), Figs, Grapes (purple), Kale (purple), Olives (black), Plums, Potatoes (purple), Prunes, Raisins, Rice (black/purple)

BENEFITS

Cancer protective, healthy inflammatory response, cell protection, cognitive health, heart health, liver health

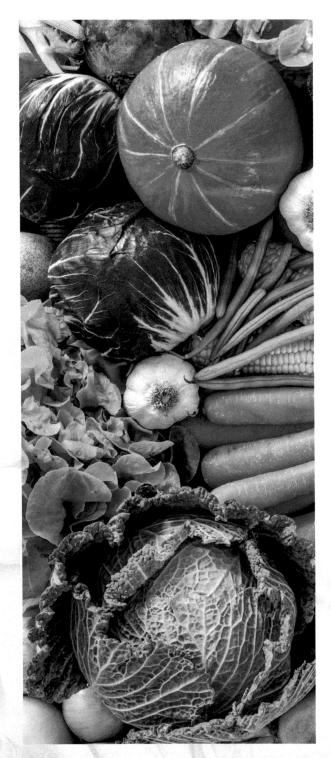

Let's engage in plant food - microbe cross-talk

A rainbow diet wouldn't have half the health impact without our gut microbiome. Rainbow plant foods provide fibre (prebiotics) that feed our diverse microbial ecosystem and ensure we cultivate within us the communities most beneficial to us. Food is also the source of many of our gut bacteria. So, the more diverse your diet, particularly in plant foods, the more diverse your gut bacteria will be.

Not only will your body thank you for eating a rainbow every day, but you'll be rewarded by a healthy, happy gut to help support and regulate all 12 body systems — including your brain.

Fresh from the farm gate

Changing the way that a plant grows, is fed or processed fundamentally changes the interaction of the naturally-occurring nutrients. This is one of the main reasons why we suggest eating organic where possible or from the 'farm gate' for freshness. Many vitamins and enzymes in plants are degraded and quite quickly lost once they're picked, so finding a source of fresh, soil-laden, plant food is preferable to pristine, plastic-wrapped veg in the supermarket. But, eating some is better than none if your only option is the latter.

Fabulous fibre

Healthy intakes of fibre have long been linked with many health benefits including a lower risk of heart disease, diabetes, obesity and bowel disease. Governments around the world typically recommend adults eat around 25-30g of fibre per day (UK, US, Australia) but many people fail to come close to recommended levels.

It's the form that matters

Unlike other carbohydrates, fibre can't be broken down by our digestive systems, but acts as food for our gut bacteria. If we don't eat enough fibre, some of the bacteria in our gut starves and dies while others grow stronger by changing their diet to feast on the mucus lining of the gut that keeps our gut wall healthy. Our gut mucosa is also the most dynamic and probably important immunological environment of our body. It's the key interface of our immune system between the inside and the outside world, and is vital to our ability to discern friends from foes, be they chemicals or organisms.

Living in the mucus layer of the intestine is a 'good' bacteria called

Akkermansia muciniphila. Recent research suggests it's one of the most important bacterial species in our gut. Among its key functions is the cleaning function it has on our mucosa, a process that generally occurs overnight, in the absence of any food. If you don't consume sufficient fibre by day, you deprive Akkermansia and other beneficial species; you promote mucus-degrading bacteria and increase the risk of gut-based diseases. In the process, you've also handicapped your immune system, your first line of attack against pathogens.

Damage to our gut environment can result in the onset of bowel issues such as inflammatory bowel disease (IBD), irritable bowel syndrome (IBS) and leaky gut leading to inflammation, a precursor to the development of chronic and auto-immune diseases.

There are of course ways of helping maintain the health of your microbiome, whilst adhering to a low carb, higher fat regime such as the Food4Health guide. One of these involves making sure you provide sufficient fibre and polyphenols, a key phytonutrient group in coloured plant foods.

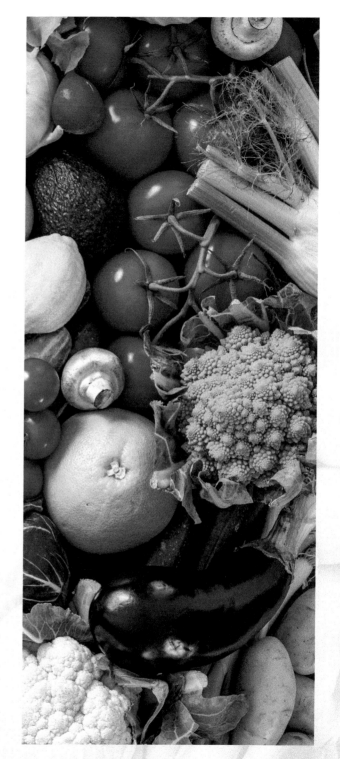

Splitting fibres

Fibre is generally classified into two types; soluble and insoluble. Both are types of indigestible carbohydrates that fulfil different functions in the digestive tract.

Soluble (prebiotic) fibre is water soluble. It dissolves in water to form a viscous gel that can then be fermented by our gut bacteria to produce short chain fatty acids (SCFAs). SCFAs help to regulate cholesterol production, improve insulin sensitivity, aid weight loss and maintenance of a healthy body weight, as well as lowering the risk of type 2 diabetes by reducing pro-inflammatory cytokines and strengthening immune function.

Insoluble fibre isn't water soluble. It adds bulk to stools to allow them to pass through the gut more quickly thereby reducing the amount of time toxins spend in the gut. Unfortunately, many of the foods we're routinely recommended to eat can cause more harm than good.

Fibre or not?

For some people, less is more! In their quest to include more fibre in their diet many people have swapped highly processed carbohydrate-based foods, such as white bread, pasta and rice for highly processed wholegrains in an effort to improve health.

The reality of this advice is a combination of a diet that's still high in one of the most common mediators of intolerance in the diet, gluten, as well as one very high in carbohydrates derived from ultra-processed grains. This combination can create a perfect storm leading to a plethora of health problems, ranging from the onset of auto-immune disease, to the acceleration of neurodegenerative conditions like Alzheimer's disease.

We recommend getting your fibre from non-starchy, above-ground vegetables in particular and in much lesser quantities from fruit. Consistent with the need to ensure a broad diversity of plants in your diet, you can choose a wide range of different plants that together help you meet your daily fibre quotient. Check out Table 4 below in which we've computed, using raw data from the USDA National Food

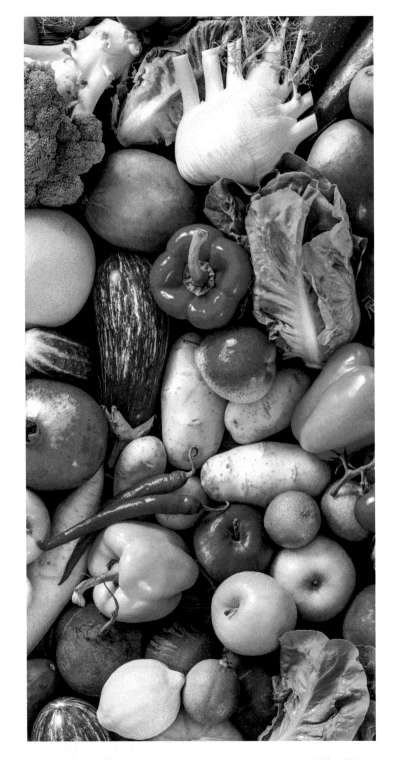

©2022 ALLIANCE FOR NATURAL HEALTH INTERNATIONAL

Composition Databases, the amounts of digestible carbs in a selection of vegetables.

And here's our big take-home point: For those choosing to follow an LCHF diet, you don't need to junk plant foods. It's still very feasible to benefit from a wide variety of plant foods assuming your body can handle them, ie. it hasn't succumbed to autoimmune related issues and can still sort out what's good for it and what's bad.

The example below (Table 4) shows just how easy it is to incorporate a range of vegetables suitable for a low carb diet to ensure the health of our gut microbiota.

To discover which foods contain different coloured phytonutrients, as well as what kind of information each of them offers your body, refer to Table 5 overleaf.

	PORTION SIZE (G)	DIGESTIBLE CARBS BY PORTION % BY E	DIGESTIBLE CARBS % BY WT	INDIGESTIBLE CARBS* % BY WT
Broccoli	60	0.72	2.21	0.60
Cabbage (red)	50	57.33	0.73	0.30
Fennel	10	28.00	0.34	0.20
Radish	25	4.40	2.74	1.30
Walnuts	20	57.00	0.97	0.40
Peppers (bell)	20	47.60	3.98	1.60
Cauliflower	20	57.33	2.09	0.80
Green Beans	30	47.20	0.99	0.40
TOTAL		**18.47**	**14.05**	**5.60**

*Indigestible carbs = fibre

Table 4. Carbohydrate composition of 8 plant foods

Table 5. Examples of phytochemicals, the foods they can be found in and some of their health benefits

PHYTOCHEMICAL(S)	PLANT-COLOUR	PLANT-SOURCE	POTENTIAL-HEALTH-BENEFITS
Carotenoids (such as beta-carotene, lycopene, lutein, zeaxanthin)	Orange, Yellow, Red	Red, orange and green fruits and vegetables including broccoli, carrots, cooked tomatoes, leafy greens, sweet potatoes, winter squash, apricots, cantaloupe, oranges and watermelon	May inhibit cancer cell growth, work as antioxidants and improve immune response Protective role against cognitive decline associated with ageing Role in protection against hepatoxicity
Flavonoids (such as anthocyanins, flavonols, flavanones)	Purple, red, blue, black	Apples, citrus fruits, onions, coffee and tea	May inhibit inflammation and tumour growth; may aid immunity and boost production of detoxifying enzymes in the body Anti-oxidative, anti-inflammatory, anti-mutagenic and anti-carcinogenic properties Cardiovascular protective
Indoles and Glucosinolates (sulforaphane)	Green, white	Cruciferous vegetables (broccoli, cabbage, collard greens, kale, cauliflower and Brussels sprouts)	May induce detoxification of carcinogens, limit production of cancer-related hormones, block carcinogens and prevent tumour growth

©2022 ALLIANCE FOR NATURAL HEALTH INTERNATIONAL

PHYTOCHEMICAL(S)	PLANT-COLOUR	PLANT-SOURCE	POTENTIAL-HEALTH-BENEFITS
Isothiocyanates (sulforaphane)	Green, white	Bok choi, broccoli, Brussels sprouts, cabbage, cauliflower, horseradish, kale, kohlrabi, mustard, radish, rutabaga, turnip, and watercress	May induce detoxification of carcinogens, block tumour growth and work as antioxidants Help with management of blood glucose, particularly in diabetic patients Helps reduce inflammation
Polyphenols (such as ellagic acid and resveratrol)	Green, Purple	Green tea, grapes, wine, berries, citrus fruits, apples, whole grains and peanuts	May prevent cancer formation, prevent inflammation and work as antioxidants Essential phytochemicals for modulating the effects of aging and promoting healthy longevity Gut protective - reduction of inflammation in inflammatory bowel disease
Terpenes (such as perillyl alcohol, limonene, carnosol)	Red, yellow, green	Cherries, citrus fruit peel, rosemary	May protect cells from becoming cancerous, slow cancer cell growth, strengthen immune function, limit production of cancer-related hormones, fight viruses, work as antioxidants Antihyperglycemic and hypolipidemic

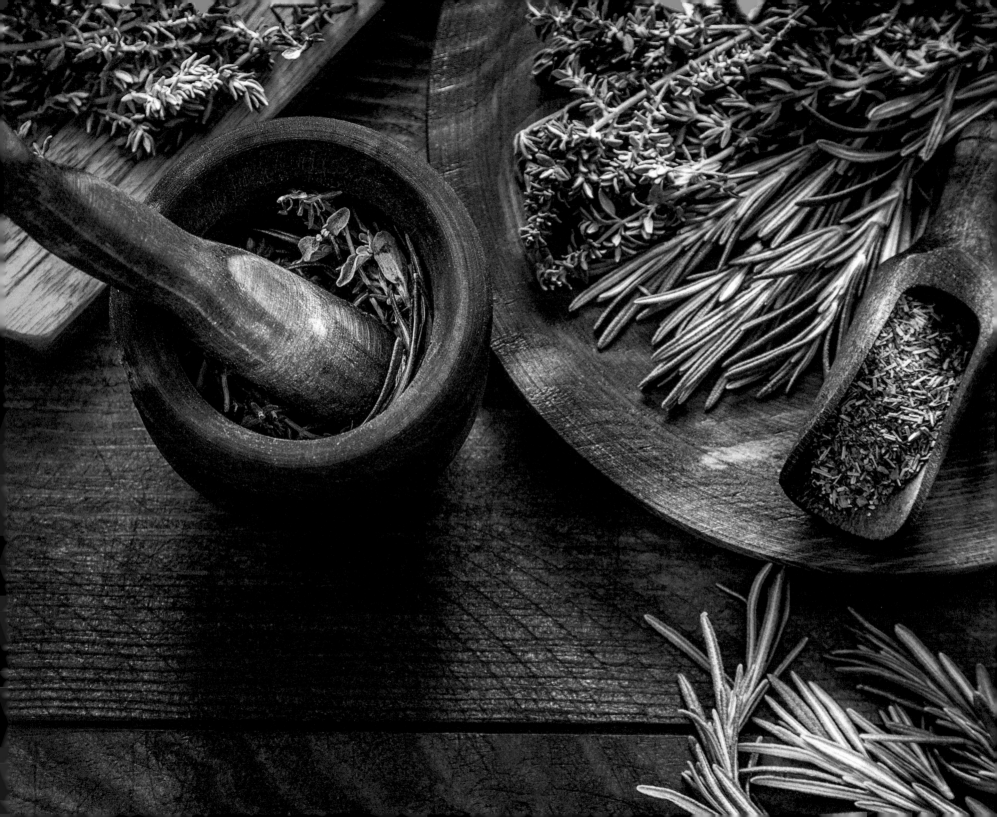

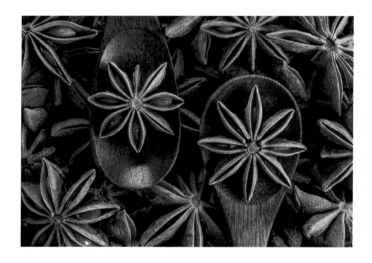

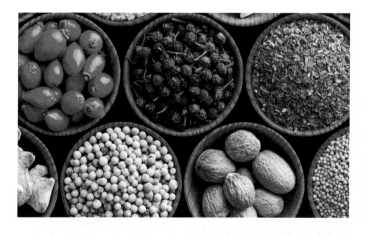

HERBS & SPICES: THE MEDICINE IN YOUR KITCHEN

We feel herbs and spices are so important in building a diverse diet that they warrant their own segment in our Food4Health Guide.

Culinary herbs used to be a mainstay of food preparation. Their use in the days before fridges was to sanitise and preserve food, assist digestion, provide medicinal benefits and prevent food poisoning. The same active compounds that were present 'back in the day' can still be found today, yet most people add herbs and spices to their food simply for flavouring purposes. Many culinary herbs found in supermarkets are also often degraded versions of their original cousins and there's an enormous difference between dried and fresh herbs and spices. Your kitchen is truly the heart of your medicine cabinet.

Herbs and spices don't just add flavour to food or beverages, they are packed with phytonutrients, antioxidants, minerals and vitamins that are essential to achieve and maintain optimal health.

Herbal history

Medicinal uses of plants have been described in writings as far back as 3,000 BC in both ancient Chinese and Egyptian texts. Indigenous cultures relied (and still rely) on medicinal plants as their first line medicine, as do traditional medicinal systems such as Ayurveda and Traditional Chinese Medicine today. This isn't unique to humans, animals have been doing the same throughout evolution. In fact, the non-nutritive, medicinal consumption of a diverse range of plant foods has been long known in our nearest non-human primate relatives, chimpanzees, bonobos and gorillas.

So powerful are their active compounds that botanicals form the basis for many of today's pharmaceutical drugs (around 75% have distant origins from plant compounds). Unfortunately, these new-to-nature molecules don't work in the same way or respect the cells of the body in the same way as nature, which is why so many drugs have such serious adverse side effects. Despite the desire to sideline and suppress natural medicine, drug companies still continue to look towards plants for new compounds.

Spice up your life!

Herbs and spices are readily available in health stores, groceries and supermarkets. The seeds and young herbs are also widely available in garden centres. Why not try growing your own on window sills, patios, veg plots or in amongst your garden borders? Fresh herbs and spices freeze well and are then always on hand to add to food, infuse as herbal teas, make oil infusions for dressings/marinades (see our Pesto and Chimichurri recipes) or dehydrate and sprinkle on food.

As with all foods, the better the quality and the optimal dosage for an individual, the more therapeutic the benefit. Be aware that most, non-organically certified dried herbs and spices have been irradiated for longer-shelf life and to destroy microorganisms and insects. This may damage the health-giving compounds, rendering them little more than flavour enhancers. Many of the active compounds

are delicate and are damaged by excessive processing, heat and light so treat your herbs and spices with respect and freeze them to keep them fresh.

Herbal teas are a wonderful alternative to caffeinated beverages and provide an amazing way of delivering water-soluble components from herbs to the body. It's a system that's been developed over thousands of years in a range of traditions, some of the most comprehensive coming out of the Indian (Ayurvedic) and Chinese medicine traditions.

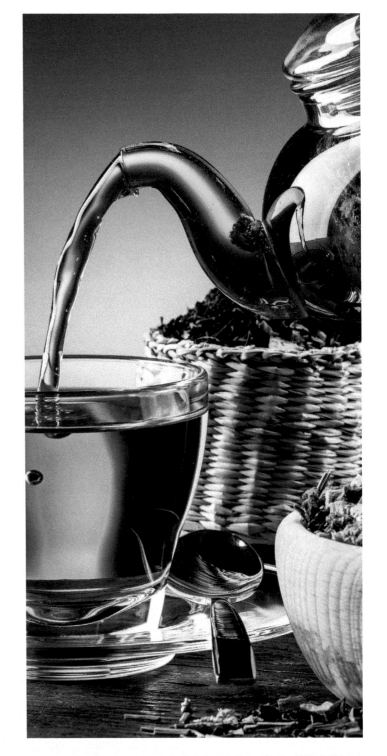

©2022 ALLIANCE FOR NATURAL HEALTH INTERNATIONAL

TURMERIC

Potent antioxidant, anti-inflammatory, anti-microbial, anti-Alzheimer, anti-tubercular, cardio-protective, anti-diabetic, hepato-protective, neuro-protective, nephron-protective, anti-rheumatic and anti-viral, anti-cancer. Use in both sweet and savoury dishes and as a supplement. Can be used either as a fresh root or dried and powdered. One of the most widely used Asian spices. Easy to drink either as a tea or 'golden milk'.

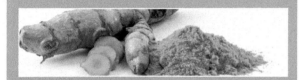

CINNAMON

One of the oldest known spices. Anti-clotting , anti-viral, anti-microbial, anti-inflammatory and blood sugar control. Use in both sweet and savoury dishes. Comes in a stick (bark) or powdered. A warming spice used in middle eastern dishes.

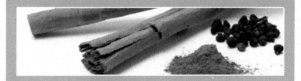

GINGER

A favourite in Asian cooking. Relief of nausea, anti-inflammatory, immune boosting. Can be used either from the fresh or dried root or powdered. Makes a warming tea and adds heat and warmth to both sweet and savoury dishes.

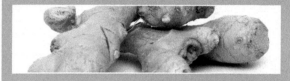

Alliance for Natural Health International presents

HEALING HERBS AND SPICES

A brief guide

Full list of references at http://anhinternational.org/2017/08/23/the-medicine-in-your-kitchen/

GARLIC

One of the oldest cultivated plants in the world. Anti-hypertensive, anti-bacterial, cholesterol lowering, cardiovascular health, anti-cancer. Best eaten from fresh either raw or cooked.

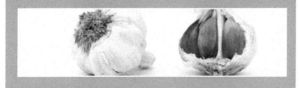

CORIANDER

A favourite in Asian dishes of all types. Anti-inflammatory, immune function promotion, antioxidant, anti-fungal. Use the leaves fresh, seeds whole or ground in both savoury and sweet dishes.

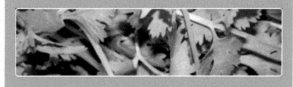

PARSLEY

Well known as a garnish or in parsley sauce! Good source of vitamin K, vitamin C, vitamin A, manganese and iron Anti-oxidant, anti-cancer, anti-bacterial. A great breath freshener, particularly after eating garlic and a great digestif.

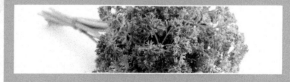

BASIL

A staple of Mediterranean cooking. Anti-microbial, anti-bacterial, anti-inflammatory, anti-cancer. Use the leaf fresh or dried. Use in sweet or savoury dishes.

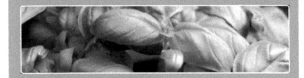

MINT

Known for its use in flavouring toothpaste and chewing gum. Anti-microbial, relieves gastrointestinal discomfort, anti-inflammatory, anti-spasmodic. Use the leaves fresh or dried or as an oil. Makes a great tea or infusion.

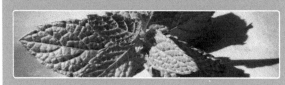

CHILLI

Used worldwide to add flavour, aroma and heat to food. Anti-microbial, anti-inflammatory, anti-cancer. There are many types of chilli from mild to WOW! They can be used fresh, dried or powdered in both sweet and savoury dishes.

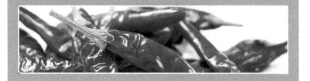

Alliance for Natural Health International presents

HEALING HERBS AND SPICES

Full list of references at http://anhinternational.org/2017/08/23/the-medicine-in-your-kitchen/

A brief guide

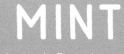

ROSEMARY

Another Mediterranean staple. Antioxidant, anti-fungal, anti-oxidant, anti-bacterial. Rosemary can be used fresh, dried or as oil. The scent of Rosemary can improve mental alertness.

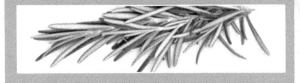

THYME

An important component of bouquet garni and herbes de provence. Anti-bacterial, anti-inflammatory, anti-cancer. Used mainly in savoury dishes, but can be used in sweet. Goes particularly well with Rosemary. Use fresh or dried.

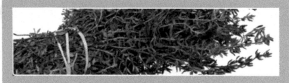

OREGANO

A staple of Mediterranean cooking along with Basil and Rosemary. Anti-viral, anti-parasitic, anti-fungal, antioxidant, anti-inflammatory, anti-bacterial. Can be used fresh or dried or as an oil.

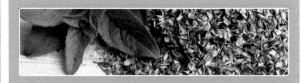

©2022 ALLIANCE FOR NATURAL HEALTH INTERNATIONAL

THE TWO MOST COMMON ALLERGENS

As a society, we are now dying slowly (mostly uncomfortably and painfully) from chronic inflammatory and metabolic diseases, not fast from acute infections as our ancestors used to. Interestingly nothing much has changed in 40 years as far as genes and environmental triggers go, yet acute chronic disease rates continue to rise. Would it surprise you to know that we're not born with the destiny to develop chronic inflammatory diseases? The stark fact is that our current health crisis is not down to genetic changes or infections (pathogens), it's down to something we are doing to ourselves and the planet.

Among the most important, known stimulators of autoimmune and chronic inflammatory diseases are gluten (the protein in wheat, barley, rye, spelt and triticale) and dairy (around 75% of the world's population can't digest lactose) which can trigger acute and debilitating gut dysfunction — resulting in traumatised gut microbes!

Removing gluten, and potentially dairy, from your diet whilst taking better care of your gut bugs are simple changes that can take you giant strides away from the edge of the disease cliff. This is why the ANH-Intl Food4Health Guide is 100% gluten-free and lists dairy as optional.

Gluten

Have you ever tried going gluten-free for more than 2 months, especially alongside healthy foods with a minimum of additives? If not, it's worth a trial and then seeing how you feel when you re-introduce it. You'll then understand completely why there is such a trend towards going gluten-free that has absolutely nothing to do with fad diets or mental health conditions!

Up until recently, most people, whether members of the public or health professionals, thought a gluten-free diet was only for the 1% or so of people diagnosed with coeliac disease. As research

progresses and results from clinical practice emerge, we now know that gluten (a protein found in some grains) and associated proteins (gliadins and glutenins) can contribute to health issues in a much wider part of the population. The spectrum of gluten-related disorders broadly spans three categories: autoimmune, allergic and non-autoimmune/non-allergic conditions.

Gluten-related disorders

Included among those affected by gluten are therefore not only coeliacs, but also people who suffer from wheat allergy (Ig-E and non-Ig-E-mediated) and those who have, what is now referred to, as Non-Coeliac Gluten Sensitivity (NCGS). First referred to in the 1980s, NCGS is the term used to describe individuals suffering a range of symptoms, not linked to autoimmune disease, that quickly improve after gluten is removed from the diet, and in which both coeliac disease and wheat allergy were properly ruled out. If gluten exposure is maintained, there is a risk that very serious conditions, such as autoimmune thyroiditis, may occur in around 1% of the NCGS population, itself difficult to estimate given the low rates of reporting and medical diagnosis.

Making matters even more complicated is the scale of under-reporting linked to gluten-mediated type 1 diabetes and cancer, both of which are triggered via autoimmune reactions. These conditions are frequently undiagnosed as being gluten-mediated and being forms of 'silent coeliac disease', they result from years, or decades, of chronic exposure to gluten.

A prevailing view among the medical establishment is that less than 10% of the population would benefit from wheat exclusion. Taking then a conservative estimate of 6% of the population being affected by gluten-related disorders, that still equates to 3.9 million Brits and 19.4 million Americans being affected, who would massively benefit from going gluten-free. And that's a conservative view! That's enough to ensure anyone suggesting gluten-free is a fad is either ignorant of the facts or they have no interest in public health.

Gluten – the silent enemy

The lining of your gut, the mucosa, has doorways along its length called tight junctions. These tight junctions act as regulators between the internal environment in the gut and the body. Vital food nutrients pass across the intestinal wall, toxins are kept out, but the 'doorways' are only flung open when the gut's defence system meets a pathogen that's too fierce for it to cope with alone. By opening the tight junctions, and therefore making the gut permeable (leaky), the body's full immune armoury can be brought to bear. It's a survival strategy that's seen us through evolution up until the present day.

A protein molecule called zonulin is the gatekeeper, opening and closing the doorways when necessary. All of this has worked well up until we were faced with gluten and diets that make our guts inflamed.

Gluten is actually not just one compound. It's a mixture of hundreds of distinct proteins that are common to cereal grains such as wheat, barley and rye. They can be loosely divided into two classes of protein: gliadin that helps bread to rise when it's baked and glutenin, that gives bread its much-loved elasticity.

In a nutshell, gluten mimics the action of zonulin and flings

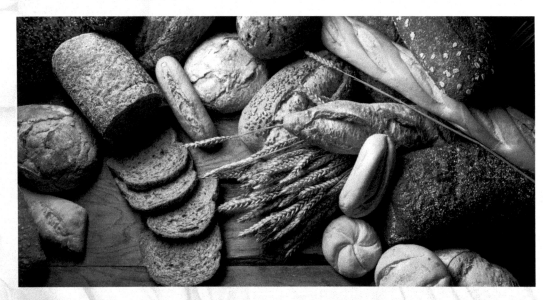

©2022 ALLIANCE FOR NATURAL HEALTH INTERNATIONAL

open the doorways of the gut mucosa thereby creating intestinal permeability or a leaky 'teabag' gut. Apart from having the gut contents flowing out into the body, so too do our intestinal microbes – whether they be good guys or bad guys – in search of new homes in our organs or worse, our brain. Both actions have consequences that cause the big guns of our body's immune system to crack down hard, causing inflammation, which underlies all of the big, chronic diseases, from most forms of cancer to heart disease, from arthritis through to type 2 diabetes or obesity.

Even worse, the immune system can get confused and start attacking some of our own cellular proteins thinking that they're enemies. Do this for a prolonged period of time and you have the 'perfect storm' that triggers autoimmune diseases, which are rising fast with over 100 now described in the medical literature.

Dairy

Governments, the food industry and the dairy marketing boards have done a great sales job. Despite around 75% of people round the globe being unable to digest lactose, a truly enviable PR and marketing campaign has managed to convince a large majority that cows' milk is the food of the Gods and must be consumed daily, especially by the young. If you're a baby calf, of course, it truly is the food of the Gods. But for human beings over the age of 5, it can be the root of much distress and ill health, though this is rarely recognised as such by mainstream medicine and public health programmes.

So ingrained are the dairy marketing campaign messages that trying to educate on the problems caused by drinking the breast milk of another mammal after weaning is akin to trying to change a conditioned world view.

However, it may not all be down to good marketing. Milk contains a naturally powerful opiate from the morphine family. Casomorphins are peptides, protein fragments, released from the digestion of the protein fraction, casein, in milk.

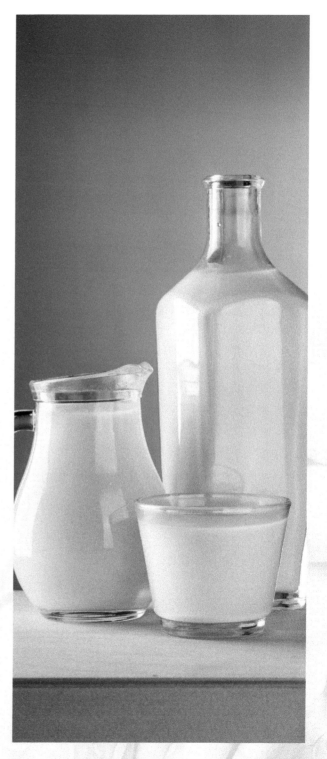

They are opioids and can have an addictive effect through mimicking the effects of opiate drugs like heroin and morphine. Once the incompletely digested peptides are absorbed into the body they bind to opiate receptors in the brain and have the power to alter behaviour and physiological reactions. So, if you've ever wondered why cheese, ice cream and milk chocolate are such comfort foods, wonder no more.

It's not just sugar that's addictive. We don't let children use heroin, yet many parents are of the mistaken belief that they have failed in their parental responsibilities if their offspring aren't drinking at least a glass a day. Milk may seem like a safe and friendly 'legal high', but it can come with a high price tag for your health.

Mother's milk

Definitely a food of the Gods for babies and even the opioid components serve a purpose. Not only do the casomorphins slow intestinal movements and have an anti-diarrhoeal effect, but they also calm the baby and assist the bonding process with mum. That's one of the reasons why babies sleep so peacefully and soundly after they've breastfed. An infant's gut also produces lactase, the enzyme needed to break down the lactose (milk sugar). But lactase production drops off steeply after weaning making lactose intolerance the most common, and well-studied, carbohydrate intolerance in the world. It's also

virtually incurable without the aid of external lactase enzymes.

The term, lactase persistence, is used to describe the ability to maintain the production of the gut enzyme, lactase, to digest lactose through adulthood. Believe it or not, it's relatively new in human evolution. Anthropologists have linked the start of animal agriculture with dairy cows and lactase persistence in both northern European and African cultures back about 10,000 years ago. In Asia, for instance, lactose intolerance is still dominant. They have a lot of cows, but not much of a history of milking them. Isn't nature amazing?

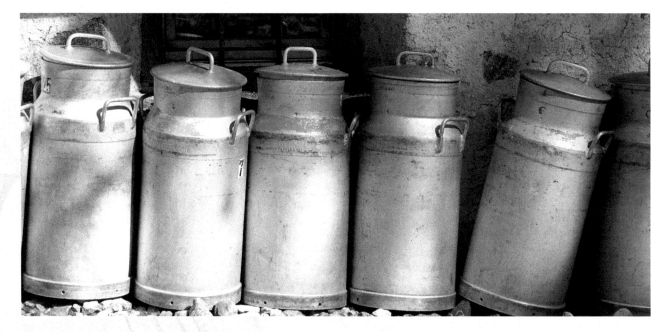

   ©2022 ALLIANCE FOR NATURAL HEALTH INTERNATIONAL

Milk and the autoimmune connection

Despite the range of nutritional factors in mammalian milk, there are still a very significant number of people, up to 100% in some ethnic groups, for whom milk represents a significant health risk, rather than a superfood. Whilst raw milk — preferably raw A2 milk — is unquestionably the healthiest and best tolerated cow's milk option, it still doesn't eliminate issues of lactose intolerance, milk protein intolerance or the link to autoimmune conditions that affect some subsets of the population. Secondary lactose intolerance, caused by impaired digestion through an imbalanced gut microbiome (dysbiosis) that affects the ability to make lactase, can also happen at any time in life.

Autoimmune disease is a broad term that applies to a diverse range of conditions with different symptoms that all have the same issue at the core. Immune cells start attacking 'self' cells as pathogenic invaders — the body literally turns on itself. The mechanism for this has been attributed to molecular mimicry where immune cells lose the ability to differentiate between self and the 'memory' of an antigen or invading pathogen.

Consumption of cow's milk, alongside gluten, leads to one of the highest levels of intolerance for the reasons already stated. But the double whammy is caused by the similarity in structure between some of the protein molecules and cells that exist in the human body. Unless you have a rock solid, healthy and impermeable gut — which is extremely rare given the prevalence of leaky gut caused by today's high dependence on gluten and wheat-based foods, some of the milk protein fractions will leak out into the surrounding tissues.

Once outside of the gut, they may trigger an immune reaction as the body reacts to the foreign proteins and starts destroying them. It's a perfectly natural process for your immune cells to then create a 'memory', which will ensure a faster reaction the next time the same occurs. It's a very effective evolutionary strategy for survival, but in those susceptible to auto-immune diseases, the immune system fails to differentiate between alien molecules and those that are intrinsic to it. Environmental factors, including diet (eg. wheat, dairy), genetic vulnerability and lifestyle may increase an individual's susceptibility to autoimmune disease.

Patients with type 1 diabetes, coeliac disease, multiple sclerosis and latent autoimmune diabetes in adults have been found to have significantly increased levels of antibodies to different milk fractions in research studies. If you operate on the 'no smoke without fire' principle, this should come as breakthrough news for those of you with an autoimmune condition or family history of autoimmune disease.

Cows' milk – driver of modern diseases?

Milk may be widely marketed, highly advertised and perennially consumed, but that doesn't mean it's healthy. Lactase persistence can now be picked up in a genetic test. It's most common in northern Europe, but still only around 25% of the world's population is able to handle the proper digestion of lactose in milk. Evolution is all about survival and reproduction – it's not necessarily about health. Unless you are starving or severely malnourished, there is actually no nutritional requirement to drink milk past infancy — and including significant quantities of cows' milk or dairy in your diet can be particularly dangerous to your health.

Here are some reasons why we've largely left milk out of the Food4Health Guide, and left it as an option to add back in:

- Milk can increase your fracture risk – according to the Nurses' Health Study, dairy consumption may increase your risk of fractures by 50%

- Milk doesn't prevent osteoporosis – interestingly countries with the lowest consumption of dairy products and calcium (Africa and Asia) have the lowest rates of osteoporosis and associated fracture risk. Around 32% or less of calcium from cow's milk is absorbed, as against 40-64% from plant foods. But calcium is far from the only player in building strong bones

- Dairy intake is linked to prostate cancer

- Dairy intake is also linked to breast cancer due to the high levels of insulin-like growth factor 1 (IGF-1) and oestrogens. Not only do the oestrogens increase the risk of breast cancer, but they also stimulate IGF-1 expression forming a vicious circle. Cows' milk can also contain added bovine growth hormone and oestrogens used to encourage rapid growth for commercial reasons

- Even modest, and certainly high, dairy intakes cause digestive problems for the 75% of the world who are lactase deficient and those digestive problems drive chronic inflammation that is central to today's chronic disease epidemic

- Milk aggravates irritable bowel syndrome, yet is often included as a key ingredient in 'medical foods' offered to those with IBS, Crohn's Disease or Ulcerative Colitis

- Milk consumption has been linked in epidemiological studies to ovarian cancers, an increased risk of autoimmune diseases, type 1 diabetes, multiple sclerosis, obesity and heart disease.

This list is by no means definitive, but we think it's enough!

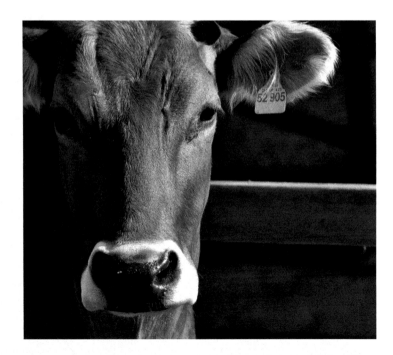

©2022 ALLIANCE FOR NATURAL HEALTH INTERNATIONAL

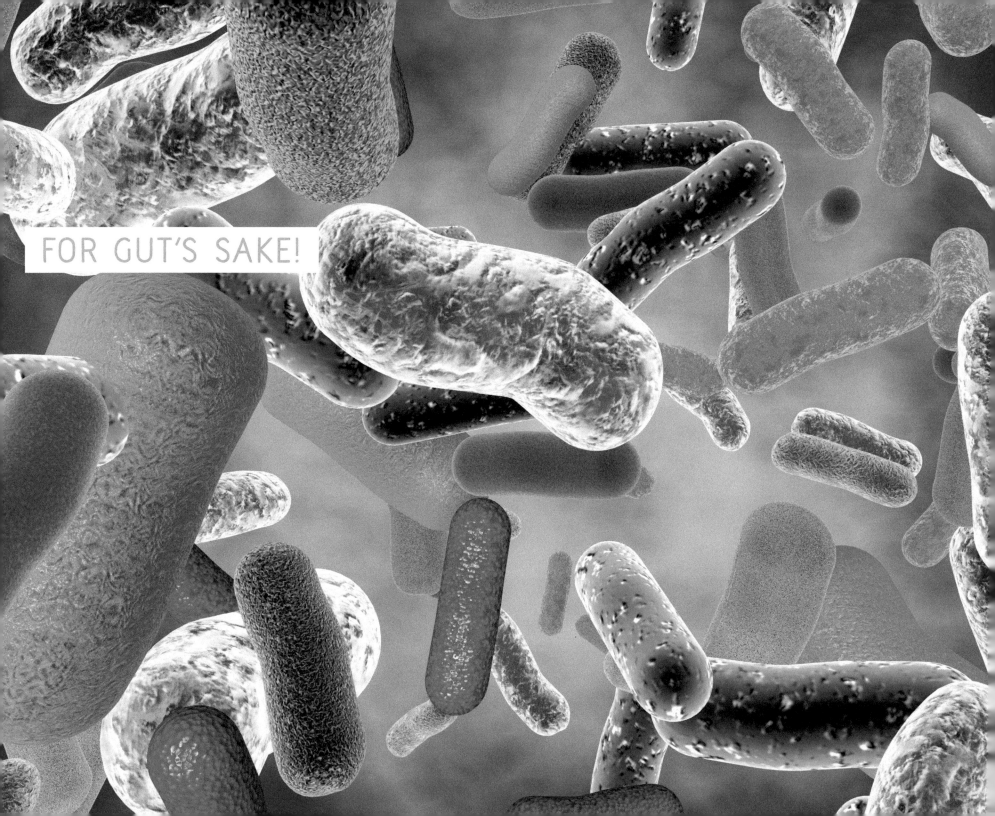

FOR GUT'S SAKE!

As an individual, you probably didn't think you had much in common with a rainforest. But you do. We all support a complex of other organisms on us and inside of us – an entire ecosystem, just like a rainforest. Throughout our evolution we humans have had an intimate relationship with an incredible array of microbes (archaea, bacteria, viruses, fungi, algae and protozoa) and helminth parasites like flukes and tapeworms. Soil bacteria, the microbes on plant matter and in animal faeces were an integral part of life – so much so that they have been literally integrated into us. It might feel slightly uncomfortable to find out that you're actually less than 1% human DNA! The rest is microbial DNA. Hence, we can't now live without them and together we make up our 'hologenome'. Talk about a co-dependent relationship!

Whilst we have microbes on our skin and hair, in our mouths and throughout our bodies, the biggest collection by a long shot inhabits our gut. A healthy adult gut harbours a complex community of around 100 trillion microbial cells, referred to as the gut microbiome. That's about 10 times the number of human cells we have in our bodies. That also means that we have 10 times the amount of non-human genetic material than we do human DNA.

Given that our brains weigh around 1.2 to 1.5 kg (around the 3 lb mark) and the biomass of our microbiome, when we're healthy and haven't disinfected ourselves with antibiotics, is about 2 kg (about 4 ½ lb), you'd be right to wonder if you're actually driving the bus. The simple answer is: no, not always!

These gut microorganisms use plant compounds that we've consumed to regulate a wide range of critical functions (transcriptomics) including our appetites, our immune systems, our brain function and the way we store and use energy. They also have a lot more to say about what drives our needs and desires ie. what we eat, our relationships and our social interactions, than we give them credit for. Even our energy generating factories within cells, the mitochondria, have evolved from bacteria and still contain genetic remnants.

Hence, in order to play our co-dependent role so it works in our favour, we have to learn what it means to be a good host. We also need to accept that we never eat alone. When we dine, we also dine with trillions of microorganisms who are often putting their needs out there more strongly than we are. That's an important reason why so many chronic diseases are linked to a disrupted gut microbiome: allergies, autoimmune diseases, many forms of cancer, skin conditions, inflammatory bowel disease, thyroid imbalance, type 2 diabetes and obesity to name a few.

©2022 ALLIANCE FOR NATURAL HEALTH INTERNATIONAL

A brief glimpse into gastrointestinal anatomy

Our gastrointestinal tract is basically a pipe that runs from mouth to exit. It takes in our oesophagus, stomach, small and large intestine, rectum and digestive organs, the liver, gall bladder and pancreas. It's meant to be a mostly sealed tube that has its own food factory and defence system with friends and partners to make it all work seamlessly. In return for a safe and comfortable home, our gut microbes are meant to help us digest our food and make nutrients (including folate, B12 and short-chain fatty acids) and other co-factors to see us through a vital, happy, healthy life.

The whole community project is policed by the gut's immune system that resides in the walls of the tube (the mucosa). But like any community, when the fabric of social society breaks down, problems start occurring. In the case of the gut, this happens when our partners and friends don't receive the right nourishment

or conditions, when the gut stays inflamed for long periods, when the mucosa loses its ability to distinguish friend from foe, or self from non-self, when the good guys turn to bad guys or when the gut starts to 'leak' its contents into the body cavity. If you can't get things back under control, mayhem and disease become the order of the day.

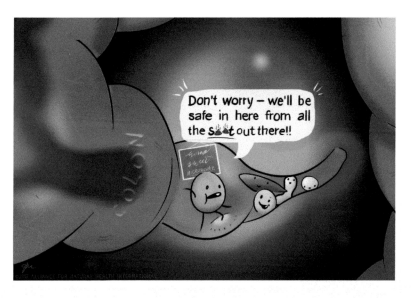

Your immune control centre

We expect a lot from the inner surfaces of our gut – the mucosa. This incredibly important interface between those elements of the outside world that we routinely put within us and our inner world, is comprised of three main parts. The outermost layer is the non-human microbiota layer that we've mentioned. Next is the highly specialised, 'intelligent' mucous layer (or layers in the case of the colon) that separate the gut contents from the innermost layer of cells of our gut, the intestinal epithelium.

The gut epithelium is one of the most biologically active areas of the body. Cells replace themselves more often than any other part of the body. Each epithelial cell might be replaced every two to five days. Compare that against an average of 8 years for a brain cell. This area is loaded with different types of immune cells that make up a veritable army to handle organisms that we, and our commensal (friendly/partner) microbes, consider to be bad for business. Examples include dendritic cells, macrophages, lymphocytes and T regulatory cells.

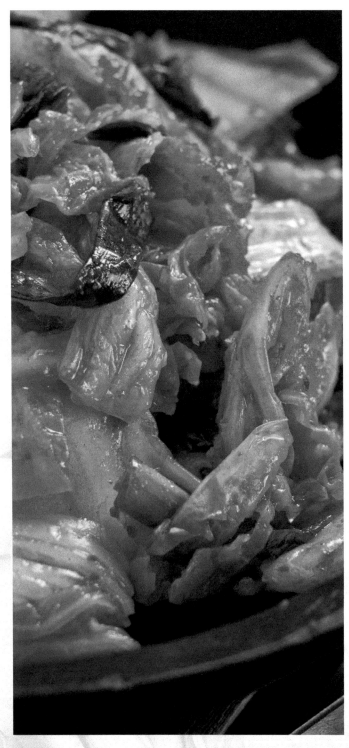

If your immune system is in balance with your gut microbiota you are the proud owner of the most sophisticated system of medicine known to our species. It's estimated that over 70% of all our immune activity goes on in our gut – that's a reflection of how important it is for us to control how we react to the outside world. Let's show some respect and also trust in the system that has ensured the survival of our species thus far.

Imagine the body's ability to identify a handful of bacteria like a pathogenic E. coli strain that might otherwise lead to a full-blown episode of gastroenteritis. Somehow the body has to distinguish these from the 2 trillion or so good bacteria – and not get confused as to what's human and not human. Speaking of E. coli – most species aren't pathogenic and there's plenty of non-pathogenic strains in our normal food, like those found in fermented foods such as miso, tempeh and sauerkraut (when it's made properly and not just pickled!)

But when the system is over-taxed, or when the function of the gut mucosa starts to breakdown or you start to experience leaky gut, the system we take for granted on a daily basis falls apart.

©2022 ALLIANCE FOR NATURAL HEALTH INTERNATIONAL

When your gut mimics a teabag

It isn't just gluten that makes our gut wall penetrable. Lectins (see the next section) can wreak havoc by damaging the gut wall, as well as other foods that trigger intolerance or sensitivity. As we've seen, gluten can fling the doors open, but the gut's defence system will open them deliberately if it feels overwhelmed and in need of help from the body's immune system. In this way, foods that trigger sensitivity and cause the creation of antibodies, can also contribute to leaky gut syndrome, much like water through a teabag. In case you're wondering, wheat, egg and dairy are the top 3 allergens.

For most people, this decline to a leaky gut is gradual over many years. Initial symptoms like mild indigestion, bloating and gas are waved off as normal until something more acute ensues, often years later. Some symptoms that your body might give you as a red flag include digestive disruption, chronic fatigue, ulcers, arthritis or joint pain, headaches, poor immune function, mood swings, depression or anxiety, memory loss, confusion, hormone imbalances and unexplained weight fluctuations. The length and breadth of that list should give you an inkling of how important our gut function is to us and more specifically why we need to be a good host to our microbial partners.

You might not be able to do anything about the genes you inherited, and you may also have been born by C-section or been formula fed in your early weeks and months. All of that means your microbiome may be compromised compared to the norm, which may make you more susceptible to a leaky gut. But the good news is you can help rebuild the integrity of your gut – especially by altering what, how and when you eat, all things that are largely within your control.

The first major step towards better gut health is to provide the plant foods, fibre and phytonutrients, like polyphenols, that not only feed our friends (prebiotics), but also ensure that we have the right ones setting up home. We hope that we've laid out a strong case for cutting out or down on refined, starchy carbs and sugar, both of which cause yeasts to flourish and the overgrowth of less beneficial bacteria in places they shouldn't be, like your small intestine (creating SIBO: small intestinal bacterial overgrowth).

Less well known is the part that food additives play in breaching our tight junctions. Choosing whole, minimally processed foods without additives and cooking at home from scratch is your best protective action for your gut.

You also need to pay attention to any not-so-good stress to which you might be exposed, especially if it's ongoing. Did you know that 90% of your feel-good, anti-depressive, hormone, serotonin, is made in the gut by your microbiome? Serotonin is also responsible for the rhythmic movement of peristalsis that moves your food through your GI tract. This is why living with constant stress shuts down your digestive system as your body prioritises the flight from the sabre-toothed tiger over your lunch. That's also why stress transformation practices like breathing exercises, yoga, meditation and mindfulness are so important as part of your overall health ecosystem.

Our gut-brain cross talk

Basic anatomy tells us that the gut and the brain are connected via the vagus nerve. It's a principal component of the parasympathetic ('rest and digest') nervous system, the side that's not under our conscious control (autonomic nervous system). Apart from being the longest nerve in the autonomic nervous system, the vagus nerve helps to regulate heart rate, blood pressure, sweating, digestion and even speaking to a certain extent because it controls the muscles of the voice box. It runs all the way from the brain stem to the stomach and intestines and supplies nerve function to the heart, major blood vessels, lungs, airways and the oesophagus. It's hugely important in our lives and sudden overstimulation can drop blood pressure, slowing the heart, causing a loss of consciousness.

It's also a two-way street that conveys information back from these organs to the brain. This brain-gut axis not only involves the nervous system, but also the endocrine and immune systems — and the gut microbiota. Interestingly, cutting the vagus nerve doesn't affect digestive function suggesting it has a 'mind' of its own. Our brain may have 100 billion neurons, but our gut has 100 million, suggesting that it really is our second brain. There's no coincidence in the fact that our microbiota, in residence within our second brain, is responsible for the digestion of foods; the creation of hormones and vitamins; response to medicine and infections; detoxification; control of blood sugar and cholesterol levels and controlling the risk of developing certain chronic and autoimmune diseases. Our gut microbes are involved in just about every process in the body, including defence.

Our health is deeply dependent on the diversity and vitality of our internal 'rainforest'. We truly are what we eat and absorb, and what happens in our gut influences how we feel, how we think, how we behave, how we defend ourselves and how we function.

It's no wonder we so value our gut feelings or experience 'butterflies' in our stomach at momentous times in our lives.

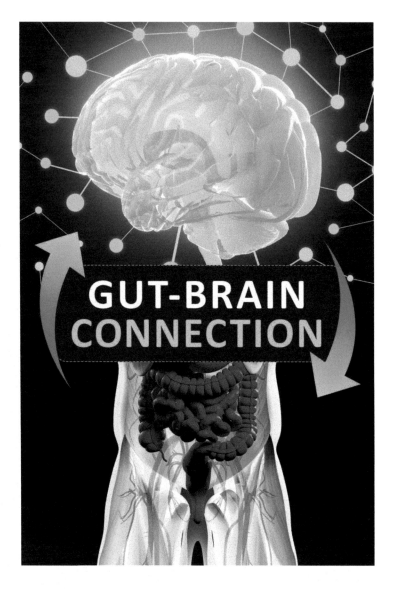

GUT-BRAIN CONNECTION

©2022 ALLIANCE FOR NATURAL HEALTH INTERNATIONAL

When food is not our friend

Unfortunately, there are certain foods which have the power to damage our gut. We have discussed why we exclude gluten from our Food4Health guidelines and the following section discusses lectins, phytates, oxalates and histamines. However, a healthy, robust gut can manage a certain amount of foods containing antinutrients. Depending on your cultural background, ethnicity and foods you've become used to, you may not experience any adverse effects at all. But if you have a sensitive gut, autoimmune disease in your family history, health or fatigue issues, try to avoid overloading your body with these foods. Peanuts, in particular, can have lectins that are problematic for many.

Vegetables and grains which cause a foam on the water as you cook them (onions, rice, potatoes, soya beans, legumes) contain saponins which can take out whole sections of your epithelial layer. But there's no need to lose them from our diet. Rinsing rice and soaking legumes (pulses; beans) overnight before cooking them rids them of most of the saponins — cooking legumes for over 6 hours can destroy the lectins too. You can speed this up if you have a pressure cooker. The reason why we have historically cooked onions on a low heat until they become transparent (before adding the other ingredients), ensures that the saponins are destroyed before you add the rest of your ingredients.

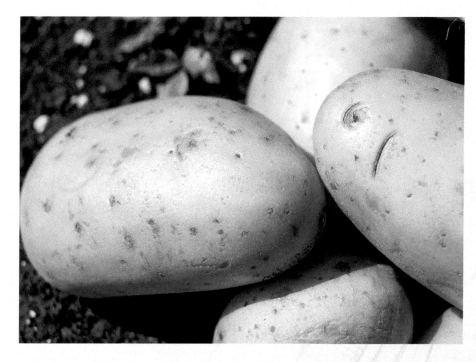
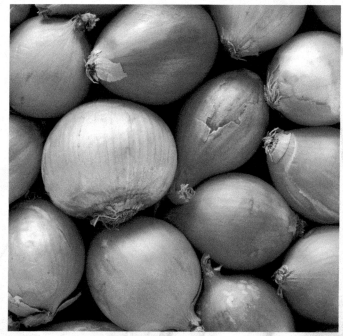

©2022 ALLIANCE FOR NATURAL HEALTH INTERNATIONAL

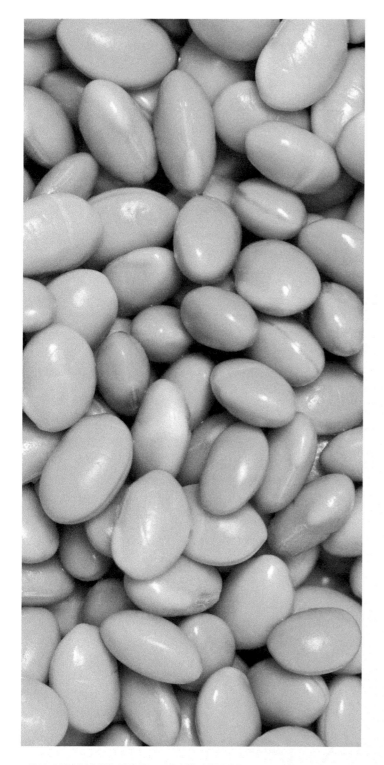

Lectins

Plants were here a very long time before humans and other animals. The first photosynthetic plants appeared on land around half a billion years ago, and flowering plants – which include the main crops we eat – around 200 million years ago. Turn that 200 million years into a 24-hour clock and you'll find we modern humans have only been around for just 90 seconds!

If you're a plant, it's been a busy time. It's way more crowded now and green plants have found themselves relegated to the bottom of the food chain, literally. But in order to survive, plants have evolved an arsenal of chemical warfare agents as part of their survival strategy. Plant lectins are one of the prime agents in that arsenal, although they're thought to have other functions in a plant too, especially ones linked to cell communication and recognition.

Plant lectins represent a very diverse family of protein molecules. One of their stand-out roles is to protect their babies from invading microbes and insects. They're referred to as 'sticky' proteins because they bind to particular sugar (carb) components on cell membranes, especially molecules called glycoproteins and glycolipids. Most plant lectins cause cells to clump together, hence the name 'agglutinin' eg. wheat germ agglutinin. Once attached to sugar molecules, they can become stealth invaders. They can hack into a microbe or herbivore's system and really mess with it.

Take for example, sialic acids. These are sugar molecules involved in cell to cell communication. When lectins bind to sialic acid, they're able to hack in and disrupt the communication between neurons and, in this way, they can paralyse an insect herbivore making it prey instead. Not being equipped to do the business themselves, the lectins release pheromones that call in the herbivore's predator to do away with it as it lies there paralysed.

Lectins are produced by all classes of living organisms and even by different types of cells. They are structurally very diverse and can have highly specific functions like

©2022 ALLIANCE FOR NATURAL HEALTH INTERNATIONAL

enzymes or antibodies. Some foods are naturally higher in lectins than others while particular lectins are more toxic than others. The other reason why lectins are called 'anti-nutrients' is because they can also significantly reduce the digestibility and absorption of protein, and some vitamins too. One of the first lessons we learn about cooking dried legumes, especially red kidney beans that are loaded with lectin phytohaemagglutinin, is that they need to be soaked and boiled before they're safe to eat. Improperly cooked kidney beans can kill you. Then again so can just a few molecules of ricin – the lectin from the caster bean plant.

To a plant, we're just another herbivore. Luckily, this is one time that size really does matter. The dose that paralyses an insect may not be enough to do us any harm at all, if we've got a robust constitution. Or it may take many years of regular, low-level exposure before we feel the effects. By then, of course, it's hard to narrow down the cause of our ills.

Our sensitivity to lectins varies a lot. Key considerations are the health of our gut and microbiome, our immune system, our age (younger people are generally more resilient), our overall level of vitality and, of course, the level of consumption. If you've ever felt bloated, windy or tender in the gut after indulging in too many edamame, it may have been down to lectin-sensitivity. Remember, the soybeans in edamame haven't been cooked long enough to lower the lectin levels. Typical symptoms of lectin sensitivity include bloating, diarrhoea, nausea and gas, all of which can lead to a leaky gut barrier over time and exposure. But the good news is that, addressed early enough, it's all reversible.

Our genomic line is about half a million years old. We were hunters, gatherers and foragers who used to have a heavily plant-based diet. This is why our genome and our microbiome are designed to recognise and communicate well with the lectins in leafy plants and some roots. It was only around 12 thousand years ago that grains and beans (legumes) became common staples. Before that time, we had no way of eating these plants in quantity as we didn't cultivate food crops or process them into edible foods. The result is that our genome and our gut microbiome can be challenged by these 'new' lectins – especially when they assault our system in quantity. Maybe not in all people all the time, but more so when you're immune challenged, chronically stressed, older or suffering gut distress.

California-based Dr Steven Gundry, one of the foremost clinicians and researchers into lectins and author of *The Plant Paradox: The Hidden Dangers in "Healthy" Foods that Cause Disease and Weight Gain* (2017), puts forward that we have only been exposed to lectins from the Americas for a mere 500 years. He cites this, along with exposure to too many grains and legumes, as being one of the drivers of the epidemic of autoimmune diseases. It's now thought that sensitivity to wheat germ agglutinin, the lectin in wheat, is another contributing factor to the rise in non-coeliac gluten sensitivity. The adverse reactions from which many suffer might not solely be down to the action of gluten on our tight junctions. In fact, Dr Gundry has been so successful in changing the health fortunes of his patients with a lectin-free diet – many of them vegans and vegetarians – that he's no longer a surgeon, preferring instead to use food and lifestyle modification as a healing modality.

©2022 ALLIANCE FOR NATURAL HEALTH INTERNATIONAL

For those of you who are, or who think you might be, sensitive to lectins, the biggest offenders are grains - particularly wheat germ agglutinin - legumes (including soy and peanuts), seeds (including cashews) and some of the much-loved members of the deadly nightshade family – tomatoes, eggplants, peppers (bell and chili), potatoes and yes, even the beloved goji berry. But all is not lost! There are a host of low lectin vegetables out there including avocados, leafy greens, the entire incredibly healthy cruciferous family (broccoli, brussels, cabbage, pak choi, kale, etc.), carrots, cooked sweet potatoes, asparagus and all berries to name a few. When it comes to soy, do as the Japanese do and make sure it's properly fermented. As more becomes known about the adverse effects of lectins, look out for companies catering to the needs of vegans with lectin-free products.

Many cultures safely navigate lectins in their diet through long cooking times (or a pressure cooker which nukes lectins, but preserves most nutrients), high temperatures (although these can degrade nutrients), fermenting or sprouting, or by pairing them with other foods.

In India, for example, it's common to eat a lot of okra alongside lentil-based dhal. Firstly, a true dhal is often slow cooked for several hours, this substantially reduces the lectin content. Secondly, the mucilaginous part of okra is particularly good at binding lectins, as is seaweed, especially bladderwrack.

Many lectins are found in the skins and seeds, so peeling and deseeding fruits and vegetables will do the trick. With legumes, think long cooking times, just like a traditional dhal. After overnight soaking and an initial fast boil for 20 mins (if using dry legmes), it takes time (up to about 6 hours) at a gentle boil to destroy these audacious chemical weapons that have stood the test of time. But it's so worth giving these foods some extra cooking love as lectins can reduce the amount of protein and essential micronutrients, like vitamins and minerals, that you could absorb from these wonderful foods.

If you're a bread lover and can tolerate gluten, opt for a traditionally fermented sourdough and let those clever microbes lower the level of both the gluten and the lectins.

Please note: a lot of supermarket sourdoughs are not authentic because they're not fermented for long enough. A good sourdough will be fermented for the traditional 24 hours.

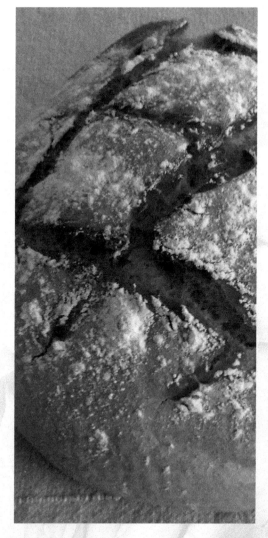

©2022 ALLIANCE FOR NATURAL HEALTH INTERNATIONAL

Phytate

Phytate or phytic acid, concentrations of which are highest in plant seeds, bran, grains, nuts, beans and other legumes, often gets a bad rap. However, like everything in nature, it's there for a reason. Phytic acid, also known as inositol hexaphosphate or IP6, is the phosphate ester of inositol. It provides the body with an important source of phosphorus and the natural sugar alcohol, inositol, helps support neurotransmitter function in the brain, as well as assisting with the binding of some steroid hormones at their receptor sites.

Its bad press comes from the fact that it has a strong ability to bind to and reduce the absorption of minerals in the gut, especially zinc, iron and calcium. That's how it's attracted the label of 'antinutrient'.

Anyone who is consuming large amounts of phytic acid-rich foods on a regular basis should be aware of its potential effects, especially on the absorption of zinc (relevant to both women and men) and iron (particularly women, who require iron in greater quantities, especially during the menstrual years). In nutritional status surveys in both industrialised and developing countries, circulating zinc levels in the blood are often found to be low, with around half the world's population considered to be deficient. This is a major issue given zinc's crucial role in modulating (balancing) the adaptive side of our immune system. It's also worth noting that zinc excess has many of the same downsides as zinc deficiency in terms of how it modulates the immune system. Therefore, trying to get the level of zinc right in the body is something of a fine art and science.

Most zinc in the West is now consumed, not from foods traditionally rich in zinc such as grass-fed cattle or wild fish, but rather in fortified breakfast cereals or in one-a-day supplements taken alongside phytate-rich breakfast cereals or bread. This impacts zinc and iron absorption.

Cooking phytic-acid rich foods, such as legumes, sprouting seeds and fermented foods (eg. sourdoughs) significantly reduces phytic acid concentrations. Consuming supplements containing zinc away from phytic-acid rich foods is another important way of ensuring the amount of zinc in your bloodstream is optimal.

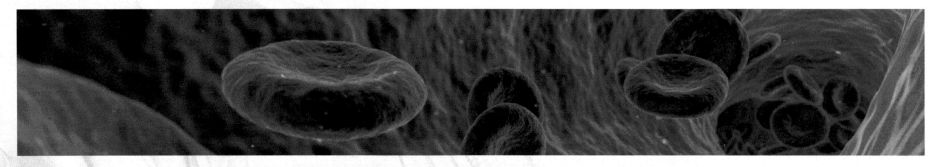

©2022 ALLIANCE FOR NATURAL HEALTH INTERNATIONAL

Oxalates and Histamines

There are another two categories about which some people need to be wary. Both are generally the result of specific conditions that develop over time and it is important that the underlying condition is diagnosed fully by a suitably qualified and experienced health professional.

Oxalates are abundant in many plant foods, especially spinach, rhubarb, nuts (and nut butters), and — wait for it — French fries and potato crisps. Therefore, vegans and vegetarians are often found to be more susceptible to high oxalate which contributes to a high risk of forming the most common type of kidney stones, calcium oxalate stones, as opposed to uric acid stones (the latter commonly associated with gout). You can readily be tested for oxalate in a blood test. If you have a tendency towards forming calcium oxalate stones, you'll benefit from eating fewer high oxalate foods and more foods rich in calcium (eg. leafy greens, legumes, amaranth).

Despite the stones being created by calcium oxalate crystals, calcium in the diet actually binds the oxalate in the gut and reduces the amount that is pushed out via the kidney and into the urine. Make sure too that you keep your magnesium intake up as magnesium has been found to inhibit calcium oxalate crystallisation.

Low-histamine diets, as with low-oxalate diets, are only relevant for those with specific health issues, in this case, histamine intolerance. One of the problems however is that histamine intolerance is often not diagnosed, and may underlie common non-coeliac adverse reactions to gluten-containing foods (ie. non-coeliac glutamine sensitivity).

Histamine intolerance is a condition in which, for one reason or another, the body produces too much histamine. This may be because the enzyme that naturally breaks down histamine produced in the body, diamine oxidase (DAO), doesn't work as it should. This can be caused by many factors such as 'leaky gut', small intestine bacterial overgrowth (SIBO), inflammatory bowel disease or particular food or drug interactions.

If this sounds like you, it's advisable that you seek help from a nutrition professional, but also stay away from high histamine foods such as: alcohol, mature cheese, all fermented beverages, avocados, eggplant (aubergine), spinach, canned and processed foods and dried fruits.

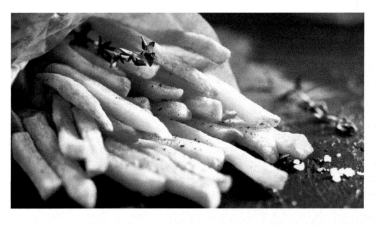

CHILDREN'S HEALTH

Re-thinking what and how our kids are eating

Our adult palates, as well as our trajectory of future health, is strongly affected by what and how we eat as children. In fact, early-life influences on our health stretch back to the time before we ingest our first solids, to pre-conception. We published our Food4Kids Guide in response to alarming global statistics for childhood obesity. Too many children are becoming metabolically derailed before they've finished developing. We owe it to future generations to change the paradigm to one of health creation.

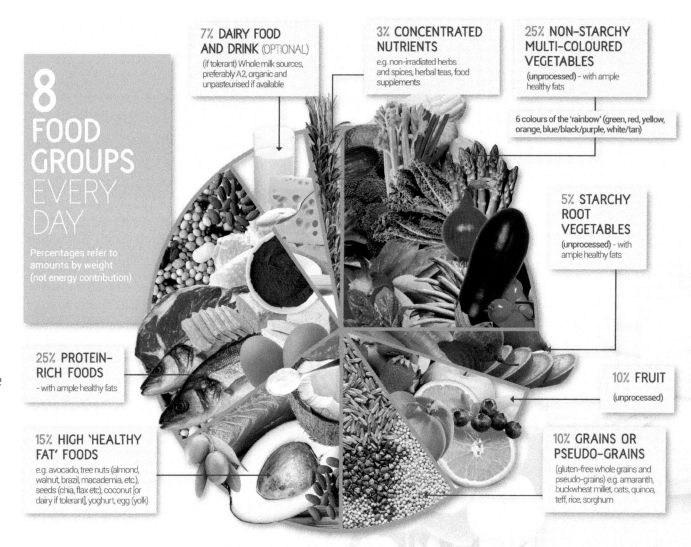

8 FOOD GROUPS EVERY DAY

Percentages refer to amounts by weight (not energy contribution)

7% DAIRY FOOD AND DRINK (OPTIONAL)
(if tolerant) Whole milk sources, preferably A2, organic and unpasteurised if available

3% CONCENTRATED NUTRIENTS
e.g. non-irradiated herbs and spices, herbal teas, food supplements

25% NON-STARCHY MULTI-COLOURED VEGETABLES
(unprocessed) - with ample healthy fats

6 colours of the 'rainbow' (green, red, yellow, orange, blue/black/purple, white/tan)

5% STARCHY ROOT VEGETABLES
(unprocessed) - with ample healthy fats

25% PROTEIN-RICH FOODS
- with ample healthy fats

15% HIGH 'HEALTHY FAT' FOODS
e.g. avocado, tree nuts (almond, walnut, brazil, macademia, etc.), seeds (chia, flax etc), coconut [or dairy if tolerant], yoghurt, egg (yolk)

10% FRUIT
(unprocessed)

10% GRAINS OR PSEUDO-GRAINS
(gluten-free whole grains and pseudo-grains) e.g. amaranth, buckwheat millet, oats, quinoa, teff, rice, sorghum

FOOD4KIDS GUIDELINES

©2022 ALLIANCE FOR NATURAL HEALTH INTERNATIONAL

Variety

Kids have notoriously different interests in foods. If not diversified and nurtured, these interests can narrow to such a degree that kids end up losing out on key nutrients they need to develop and grow healthy bodies, brains, bones, muscles and nervous systems. This can happen through the impairment of cognitive function that allows us to select healthy foods, and there is now irrefutable evidence that sugary and fatty foods affect regions of the brain in such a way as to trigger addiction. This is particularly the case in times of stress, and that is why such foods have become known as 'comfort foods'.

One of the most important roles of a parent as food provider is to help foster a broad 'palate' and healthy cognitive responses that ensure the child, and future adult, develops a strong interest in a diversity of foods able to deliver a wide range of nutrients to the body. Equally, it's critical to ensure, at the same time, that addiction to unhealthy food groups, especially sugary foods, is avoided.

Learning about healthy eating

The Children's Food Trust in the UK has undertaken research that shows there are many things that both parents and schools can do to help kids to develop a healthy approach to eating. These include:

- Laying the table; helping kids to develop a healthy approach to eating in the dining room, as opposed to in the lounge in front of a TV or on the move

- Empowering kids with cooking/ food preparation skills

We also propose:

- Allowing kids to select foods for purchase and helping them to understand their provenance (where the food originates)

- Encouraging kids to develop and design menus, based on healthy eating principles

- It is important that healthy eating habits are developed and instilled before the age of 5 so that they become habitual and are carried into adolescence and adulthood.

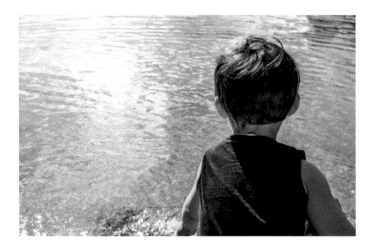

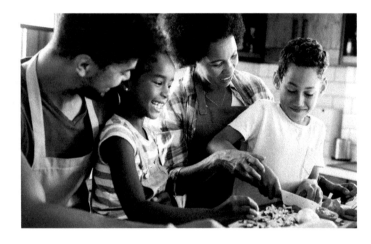

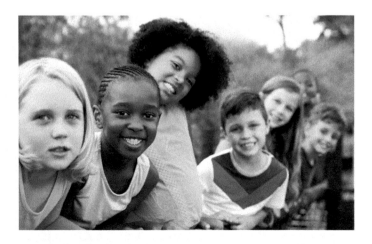

©2022 ALLIANCE FOR NATURAL HEALTH INTERNATIONAL

Sugar not so sweet!

Liquid sugar delivery system made from genetically modified corn. Rots your teeth. For anyone still driving old school cars, it's the best carburettor cleaner out there.

Also great topical medicine for leg ulcers - and for cleaning old coins. Drink it and you can get addicted.

Is it really the solution to HAPPINESS?

A public service announcement from the Alliance for Natural Health International

How much?

We are all endowed with complex signalling systems that help to regulate the amount that we eat. The problem is that this system becomes dysfunctional if we move away from a balanced and varied diet and rely heavily for our energy requirements on fast-burning, refined carbohydrates, especially sugars. This is of course the biggest challenge for kids – given the addictive capacity of sweet foods that, for the majority of our evolution, were hard to find. Now, we can walk into a supermarket, newsagent, garage – or simply open the refrigerator – and find concentrated sources of calorific, nutrient depleted foods.

Therefore, if we provide children with a diversity of foods containing sufficient proteins and healthy fats, which are especially good at signalling satiety (feeling full), along with complex carbohydrates from vegetables and fruit, children tend to regulate the amount they eat very well. They develop eating patterns that greatly reduce their risk of developing metabolic diseases like obesity and type 2 diabetes as well as tooth decay, both of which are escalating rapidly among children and adolescents.

Sugar

Most kids eat far too much sugar. For example, kids aged 4-10 in Britain consume as much as 60 g of sugar per day, a large proportion of this being in soft drinks and cereals. For teenagers it's even worse, at 74 g. While some of this sugar occurs naturally in fruits and milk, much of it is added sugars – and hidden sugars in processed and ready-made foods. A single, large vanilla milk shake, for example, from McDonalds, contains a whopping 72 g of sugars. A 330 mL can of Coke contains 35 g. These high levels of sugars are not only rotting kids' teeth at an unprecedented rate, they are also contributing to metabolic disease like obesity, at an ever-younger age.

Even the government advice in the UK is to make sure that ('free') sugars (ie. sugars that aren't naturally contained in whole, unprocessed fruit, or milk), should not exceed 5% of the energy in a daily diet. That's just 25 g total added free sugars per day for a 2000 kcal daily energy intake, well below the 35 g in a can of regular Coke.

How often

A breastfeeding infant may typically need to feed every four hours, such is their nutritional requirement. This same feeding frequency generally continues through infancy and into childhood, although increasingly it is built around 3 main meals, breakfast, lunch and dinner, with lighter snacks in between. While this is fine, and in fact wholly appropriate for a developing, growing body — for kids who are gaining excess weight, the amount of sugars and the frequency of eating are areas that need careful review. Limiting snacks in between meals is one of the most effective ways of dealing with this issue, as is ensuring that such snacks contain limited if no added sugars (see our recipe ideas at the end!).

What to eat

Healthy eating advice supported by governments normally partitions food into groups:

1. Fruit and vegetables

2. Starchy carbohydrates

3. Meat, fish, eggs, beans and other non-dairy protein sources

4. Milk and dairy products

Government authorities recommend that typically half the energy (calories) comes from carbohydrates. Our guidelines, by contrast, which are consistent with what we know of our evolutionary background, propose that only 35% of energy is derived from carbohydrates, as few of these coming from added sugars as possible, with a protein level set at around 1.2 g per kg body weight and healthy fats contributing the most to daily energy, at around 60%.

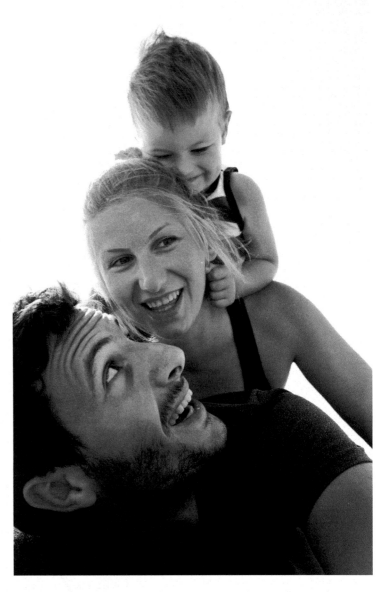

©2022 ALLIANCE FOR NATURAL HEALTH INTERNATIONAL

Food groups for ages 4 to 8

Our Food4Kids guidelines double the number of key food groups that need to be taken into account, as follows:

1. Non-starchy vegetables

2. Starchy vegetables

3. Fruit

4. Gluten-free grains

5. High animal or vegetable protein sources

6. Healthy fats

7. Milk and dairy products

8. Concentrated nutrients (e.g. fresh herbs, spices, Omega-3 essential fatty acids, vitamin D3)

The biggest challenge with balancing a child's diet according to, say, the UK Eatwell plate or the US MyPlate using these food groups is the excess of refined carbohydrates and sugars that can so easily be consumed.

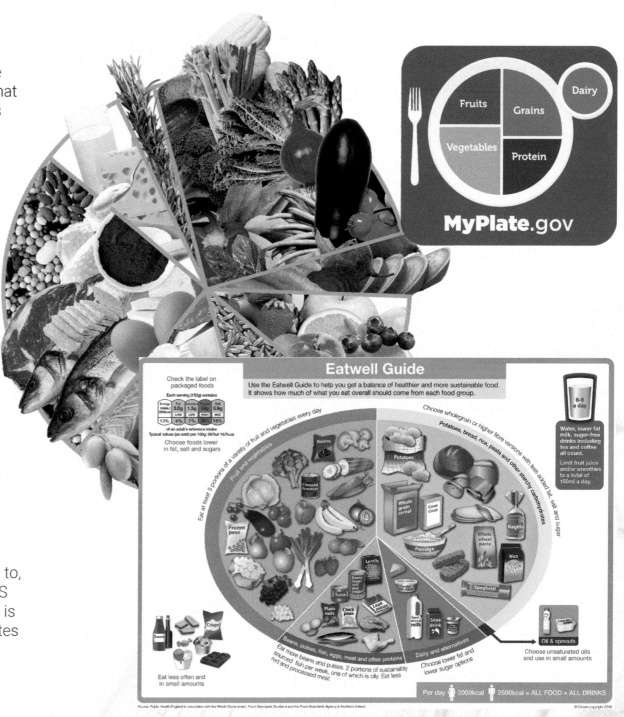

The 10 Food4Kids guidelines

A balanced and varied daily diet for infants, children and teenagers can be achieved using the following guidelines and adjusting amounts, portion sizes and meal frequency according to the age, size, gender, activity level, and cultural and other requirements of the child(ren):

1. Getting the 'macros' (protein, carbs and fats) right for young, growing bodies is absolutely key - as are the micronutrients that feed vital information to over 130 metabolic pathways essential to life. About 10% of the energy (calories) your child eats should come from quality protein, 35% from complex (not refined) carbs and around 55% from healthy fats. That fat level might sound like a lot of fats for a child, but remember that fats provide the body with over twice the amount of energy compared with either proteins or fats. [Remember: 1g of protein and carbs delivers 4 kcal (calories), while 1g of fat delivers a whopping 9 kcal]. A lot of people struggle with knowing if the protein they're giving their child is sufficient. The easy way of working it out is according to your child's body weight; for children over 1 (and up to 18), they benefit from about 1.2 grams of protein for every kilogram of body weight. Most of the weight of any given protein source is normally water or carbs, so also remember to check a nutrition calculator (e.g. the USDA's FoodCentral database, www.fdc.nal. usda.gov or NutritionValue.org).

By way of example; let's take an active 1- to 3-year-old that should be eating around 1200 kcal of energy per day (with a single main meal representing say 500 kcal of energy). The suggested daily intake of 10% protein as energy represents 120 kcal of protein for the day which simply needs to be divided by 4 to give you the actual protein content, i.e. 30 grams of protein. If all of that was to come from, say, some baked salmon (that is about 25% protein), that would mean eating over the course of a day 125 grams of the baked salmon which is equivalent to one typical boneless fillet. The reality is that your child will often be eating protein from other sources during the course of the day, which might represent the protein in half the salmon fillet (about 60 grams). This means that just half a salmon fillet would, for example, suffice for a single meal. That's equivalent to the protein in a single, large egg or 75 grams of tempeh.

2. A rainbow every day. Each day, children should consume a 'rainbow' of plant nutrients from whole fruit and vegetable sources, containing no added sugars, that includes all six colour groups, namely red, orange, yellow, green, blue/purple/black and white/tan/brown. These levels of intake will ensure that required fibre levels (which should range from around 20-40 g per day, depending on gender and age) are maintained in the diet.

3. Avoid/minimise 'free sugars. Children should not consume more than 5% of their total energy each day from 'free sugars', which include all sugars except those naturally contained in whole fruits. Fruit juices are not counted as whole fruits and are a major source of sugar in the diet and so consumption should be minimised or avoided where possible. Carbonated (fizzy) beverages (soft drinks) are among the greatest contributors to sugar intake in children and should be avoided. Be mindful of hidden sugars in sauces, salad dressings, biscuits, etc.

©2022 ALLIANCE FOR NATURAL HEALTH INTERNATIONAL

4. Drink water, not soft drinks or fruit juices. Water needs to be consumed regularly (typically 1-2 litres daily, depending on age, weight and level of physical activity) to avoid dehydration and is best consumed away from meals to avoid dilution of enzymes in the gastrointestinal tract.

5. Avoid drinks sweetened using non-nutritive sweeteners. Avoid regular consumption of intensely sweetened drinks that are either artificially sweetened (e.g. with aspartame, sucralose, acesulfame potassium, saccharin) or sweetened with natural sweeteners (eg. steviol glycosides, polyols) as these may also induce insulin resistance and confuse our cognitive and reward behaviours.

6. Avoid all ultra-processed and refined foods, especially carbohydrate-based ones or ones containing hydrogenated or trans fats. As far as possible, prepare foods from scratch using wholefood ingredients, engaging the children in the food selection, preparation, serving and tidying up process.

7. Gluten-free whole grains. Where grains are consumed, these, as with the adult plate, should be gluten-free whole grains (eg. rice, quinoa), given the prevalence of intolerance to gluten and the unknown status of sub-clinical intolerance among children.

8. Check for dairy intolerance. If there are any suggestions of intolerance from dairy foods or drinks, all forms of dairy should be avoided. Seek advice from a nutritionist or other suitably qualified and experienced healthcare professional to establish any food intolerances and to ensure adequate substitution of nutrients. Bear in mind, lactose intolerance may develop during childhood and is common in certain ethnic (eg. Far Eastern) groups.

9. Avoid heat-damaging or charring foods as excessive heat damages proteins and some heat-sensitive healthy fats (eg. extra virgin olive oil) and introduces harmful (potentially carcinogenic) chemicals such as heterocyclic amines and polycyclic aromatic hydrocarbons.

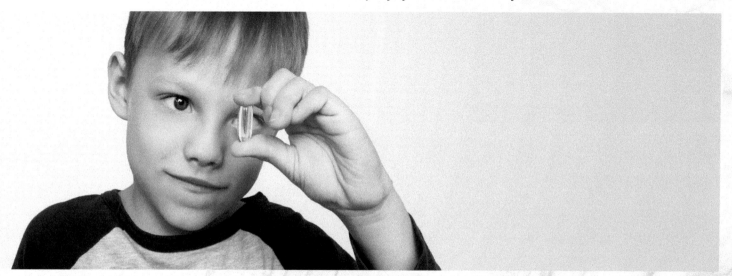

10. Include concentrated nutrients in the form of fresh (or good quality, non-irradiated) herbs and spices, along with some supplements, which may include vegetarian protein sources (especially for vegan/vegetarian children) and a limited range of food/dietary supplements, including:

- Vitamin D3 (25 mcg [1000IU])/day, from 1 month to 18 years) except when exposing around 80% of your body's surface area to the sun for at least 20 minutes of sunlight exposure

- Children's multi-vitamin/mineral (without sugar, sweeteners, fillers or artificial ingredients), as per directions

- Omega-3 oil; including EPA and at least 200 mg DHA daily (especially on days when oily fish is not eaten)

- Probiotics, from fermented foods (e.g. sauerkraut, tofu, tempeh, kimchi, etc) or good quality supplements, as per recommendation by nutritionist, other health professional or manufacturer/supplier.

©2022 ALLIANCE FOR NATURAL HEALTH INTERNATIONAL

Example: Healthy eating for a six-year old

We provide below a typical scenario of what a day of healthy eating according to the our Food4Kids guidelines might look like. For children younger, or older, amounts can be altered proportionally according to weight (refer to your country's standard growth charts for boys and girls). It is important, especially with children, to not be too prescriptive given variations in cultures, genetics, levels of physical activity and preferences. Therefore, it must be stressed that the following is simply an example of one day's eating for a typical six-year-old girl or boy, and different foods should be consumed on different days.

CARBOHYDRATES

2 cups non-starchy (e.g. mixed, coloured vegetables)(15 g carb, 60 kcal)	0.5 cup starchy carb grain (e.g. red quinoa, brown rice) (15 g carb, 60 kcal)	0.5 cup starchy root vegetable (e.g. sweet potato) (30 g carbs, 7 g sugars, 120 kcal)	1 medium banana (27 g carbs, 14 g sugars, 108 kcal)
1 apple (Granny Smith) (23 g carbs, 16 g sugars, 92 kcal)	1 cup raspberries (7g carbs, 3 g sugars, 28 kcal)	1 teaspoon maple syrup = 5 g sugars/carbs (20 kcal)	+5 g sugars from 120 g of whole Greek yoghurt (20 kcal)

Total energy from carbs = 508 kcal

PROTEIN

25 g protein total, from:

82 g red meat (150 kcal)
or 84 g chicken breast (130 kcal) (= 1 small chicken breast)
or 90 g lamb chop (150 kcal)
or 98 g (small) fillet of wild Atlantic/Alaskan salmon (180 kcal)
or 25 g pea protein isolate (100 kcal)

Total energy from protein = 100 kcal
(Total energy from high protein sources = 100-180 kcal)

FATS

Half an avocado (15 g fat, 135 kcal)
1 tbsp nut - if not allergic (eg. almond, cashew, not peanut) butter (16 g, 9 g fat) (81 kcal)
10 tree nuts (e.g. almonds, macadamia, cashew) (~6 g fat, 54 kcal)
Omega 3 DHA/EPA 0.6 g (minimum daily intake) This may be derived from as little as 28 g of mackerel, 34 g of Atlantic or farmed salmon, 38 g of tuna or 54 g of herring (but would require 200 g of cod!) (5 kcal)
Butter, preferably organic – 2 tbsp (22 g, 198 kcal)
Extra virgin olive oil (unfiltered) – 1 tbsp (13.5 g, 120 kcal)
Extra virgin coconut oil (odourless is available commercially) for cooking – 2 tbsp (27 g, 243 kcal)
Whole milk, live culture Greek yoghurt, 120 g serving (6 g fat) (54 kcal from fat, 116 kcal total)

Total energy from fats = 890 kcal

TOTAL ENERGY INTAKE = 1498 kcal (34% from carbs, 7% from protein and 59% from fats)

TOTAL SUGARS INTAKE = 50 g, with only 5 g 'free sugars' (from maple syrup)

Note: the above foods should be cooked carefully and slowly using healthy fats (see right) and fresh herbs and spices

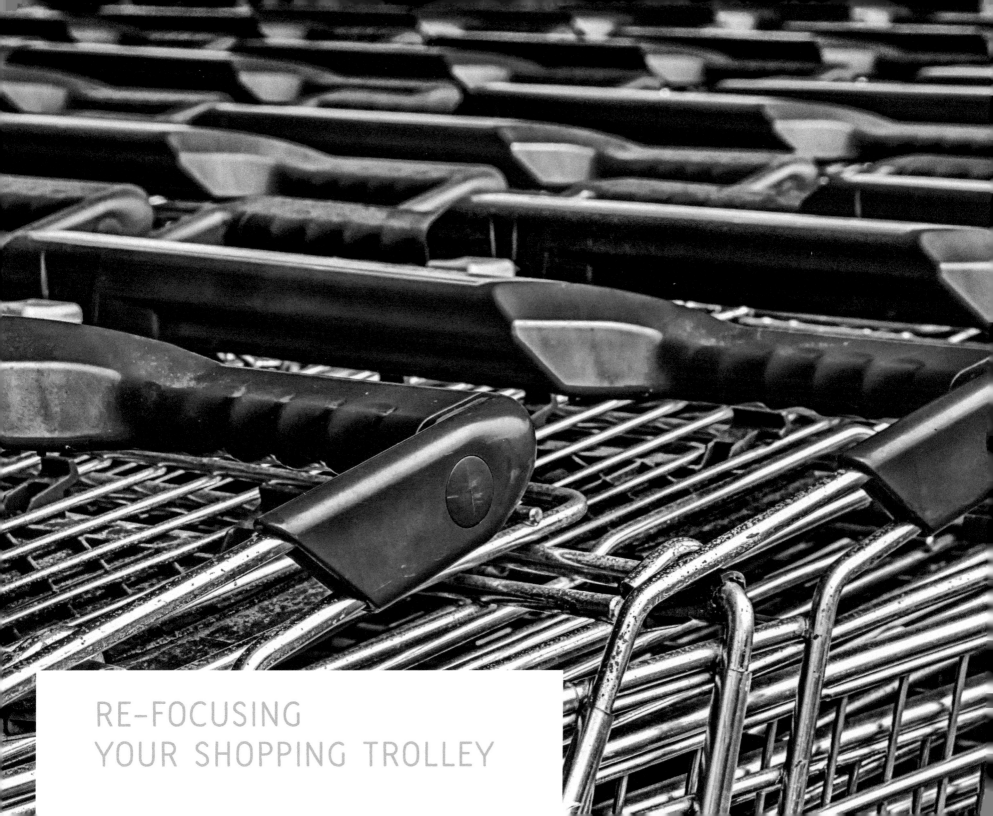

RE-FOCUSING
YOUR SHOPPING TROLLEY

Sourcing quality ingredients

What you eat is as much about what particular foods you decide to eat, as well their individual and combined quality. Less important is the quality of foods in a single meal, it's much more about the quality of food in the long-term — over weeks, months and years. So, having the occasional bit of junk food has little impact on your health — assuming that most of the time you're putting quality food into your system.

So now that we're thinking quality and long-term patterns, let's consider the places you get your food from. Here it's useful to break your food sources into 3 main groups, and recognise that as soon as you move away from cooking from scratch at home, you have less control over the quality of the food you eat:

- **Food you make from scratch in your home**

- **Food you make in your home from ready-made ingredients, sauces, condiments or other foods**

- **Foods you eat outside your home**

DECREASING CONTROL OVER FOOD QUALITY

processed ingredients and foods away from home.

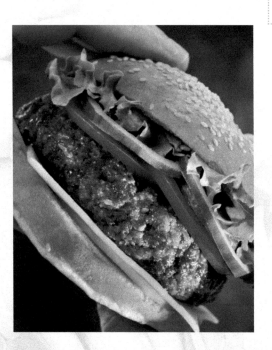

That doesn't mean that eating out will always mean you have low quality food, but it's much harder to know what you're eating. For people who eat out a lot this can be a big problem. While the Mediterranean diet is widely recognised as being a healthy diet — partially because it's one of the most studied healthy dietary patterns — there is a growing epidemic of obesity in many Mediterranean countries. More and more evidence points to this being linked to consumption of more

©2022 ALLIANCE FOR NATURAL HEALTH INTERNATIONAL

Following is our top 10 list of pointers that will help you when sourcing healthful foods:

1. **Whole foods and ingredients.** Make sure as much of your food as possible is made up of whole, not pre-processed, and especially not highly processed, ingredients. If you buy your foods in a supermarket, spend most of your time in the whole, fresh food section and avoid the aisles with processed or ready-made foods. You might want to try going bar code free for a month to get into the swing of it!

2. **Soil-grown, where possible.** Base your diet on vegetables that you know have been grown in soil, rather than in hydroponic systems. Much of the bagged, non-organic salad vegetables found in supermarkets have never seen soil. Depending on what country you live in most, if not all, organic plant foods, are soil-grown. In the EU, it is now mandatory to ensure all organic plant foods are soil-grown. But there are also many non-organic growers who continue to grow in soil, although it is harder to find out how such plants are grown and if pesticide use is avoided or minimised.

3. **Local or regionally sourced, and seasonal.** Try to consume foods that are locally or regionally sourced and in season. Otherwise you might be eating foods that have been harvested early, transported across the globe and force ripened with chemicals.

4. **Go colourful and tasty.** If the vegetables and fruit you buy are bland in colour and taste, the chances are they haven't been able to develop the full complement of nutrients (secondary compounds) they are genetically programmed to be able to produce. Having a diversity of these secondary compounds is crucial to any healthy diet.

5. **Be oil and fat aware.** One of the big drivers of systemic inflammation in our bodies is our over-consumption of highly processed vegetable seed oils along with refined carbohydrates. When you buy ready-made foods, have a careful look at the ingredients list and avoid products that simply list 'vegetable oils', especially if they also state these are 'hydrogenated' or 'partially hydrogenated'.

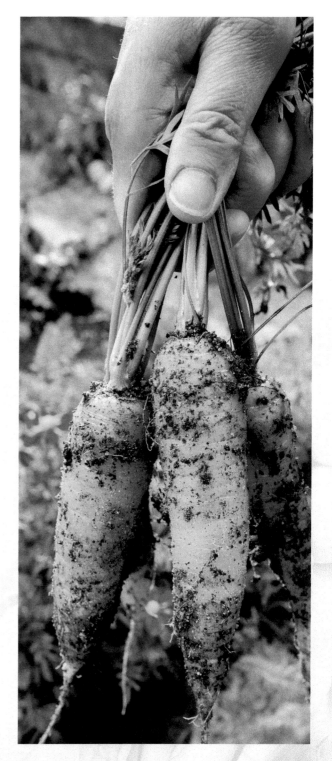

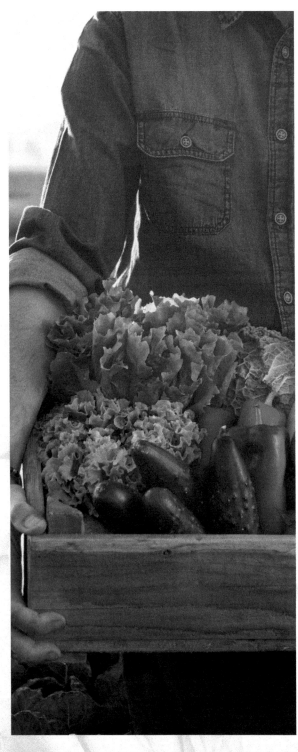

You'll find out more about healthy fats in **Macronutrients 2. Fats.**

6. **Pasture-raised / free-range livestock.** If you eat red meat, focus on sourcing your meats locally and regionally, making sure they are pasture (grass), rather than grain, fed. Meat sourced from pastures is often not only lower in pro-inflammatory arachidonic acid (an Omega 6 fatty acid), it is also more likely to be carbon neutral.

7. **Sustainably sourced.** There are an increasing number of certifications and marks that tell you something about the sustainability criteria met by the foods you eat. These include Organic, Fair Wild, Fair Trade, Marine Stewardship Council (MSC).

8. **Short, transparent supply chains.** More and more foods come from long, non-transparent supply chains, all of which add cost and make it harder for you to know what you're really eating. If you know the farm that your food ingredient comes from, all the better. If the supplier of the food doesn't know anything about the supply chain, it might be better to avoid the food.

9. **Ethos of your food suppliers.** If the supplier of your food doesn't tell you anything about their ethos, and how this relates to the health of human beings or the planet, take a wide berth. You want to try to get most of your food from responsible suppliers who're prepared to nail their principles to their front door. Some of them might even be able to demonstrate this with additional certifications, such as B Corp.

10. **Eating out protocol.** Try and find out-of-home food suppliers, whether a restaurant, take-away, snack bar or café, that can tell you exactly what ingredients are in the food or where key ingredients come from (where they were grown or raised). This is information that gives you a clear indication of food quality. Full ingredients listings are often available if you ask for the allergens listing for menu items.

   ©2022 ALLIANCE FOR NATURAL HEALTH INTERNATIONAL

Ultra-processed food dangers - cooking from scratch

Take a trip through any supermarket and you're likely to be dazzled and seduced; bombarded by the seemingly unlimited choice of ready-to-eat, drink or plastic-wrapped products. Food manufacturers have mastered their art and know just how to draw us in, pushing foods in their whole state to the very margins. As our reliance on ultra-processed foods has grown, many of us appear to have lost touch with our food, cooking less from scratch, while becoming ever more addicted to food that's not really food. As with all addictions, it comes at a price, with a swathe of non-communicable, chronic, diseases spiralling out of control.

What is ultra-processed food?

Unknown as little as 50 years ago, ultra-processed foods now make up a big part – sometimes the majority – of our diets and the foods on our supermarket shelves. These are products that began innocently as natural foods or their constituents, but have gone through multiple industrial processes and have been pumped full of additives such as colours, preservatives, sweeteners, sensory enhancers – but generally little in the way of nutrients. Many ultra-processed foods attempt to imitate the foods from which they originated, but more often than not they are far removed in terms of their nutritional composition and profile.

It could certainly be argued that the vast majority of the food most people eat each day is processed in some way or another. However, there is a huge difference between minimally processed nutrient-rich foods used for cooking or food preparation in the home kitchen as compared with the industrial-scale processing methods that result in ultra-processed foods.

The two top take homes are that:

1. **the more you process foods, the more you damage and distort them.**

2. **the more ultra-processed foods you eat, the less nutritionally balanced foods you eat.**

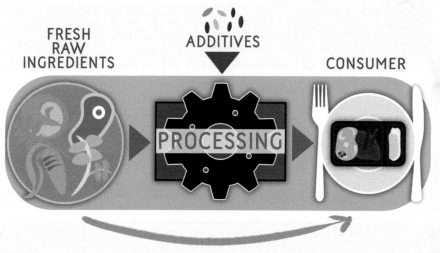

FRESH RAW INGREDIENTS — ADDITIVES — PROCESSING — CONSUMER

©2018 ALLIANCE FOR NATURAL HEALTH INTERNATIONAL

Where's the harm?

Alongside the fact that ultra-processed foods generally have limited nutritional benefit, they also contain the potential to wreak havoc on your health - and the list of possible risks is a long one.

When you manufacture ultra-processed foods, nutrients like vitamins are often lost, the profiles of fatty acids are distorted and proteins are denatured. Complex carbohydrates comprised of long glucose chains are broken down into mono- and di-saccharide units that are sugars and cause our blood sugar levels to spike each time we eat them. This increases our risk of insulin resistance and both type 2 and type 3 diabetes (Alzheimer's disease).

Many starchy carb snacks are fried or baked then covered with a cocktail of addictive additives and flavourings that have us wanting more. These seemingly delicious snacks that may have been extruded (heat treated) at unimaginably high temperatures are often high in nasty sounding chemicals like acrylamides and polycyclic aromatic hydrocarbons, both of which are known to increase cancer risk. These are just a few examples of a much further reaching problem that is impacting our diets and undermining our health with each coming day.

The International Agency for Research on Cancer (IARC) has labelled processed meat as carcinogenic to humans after finding sufficient evidence that the risk of colorectal cancer can be increased by as high as 18% daily! Highly refined carbohydrates and added sugars contribute to weight gain and obesity. Additives such as emulsifiers, organic solvents, microbial transglutaminase, gluten and nano-particles are regularly used by the food industry, rather ironically, to improve the seeming quality of their product. Despite the claims otherwise, these substances have repeatedly been linked to health issues such as allergic reactions, leaky gut, autoimmune disease and cancer. Also, damaged and trans fats have been attributed to cardiovascular disease and type 2 diabetes. If that wasn't enough, a diet high in ultra-processed foods has also been shown to promote inflammation and damage to the immune system.

Still feeling up for that plastic or foil wrapped ready-made snack? Or are you feeling the pull to rekindle a stronger relationship with your kitchen?

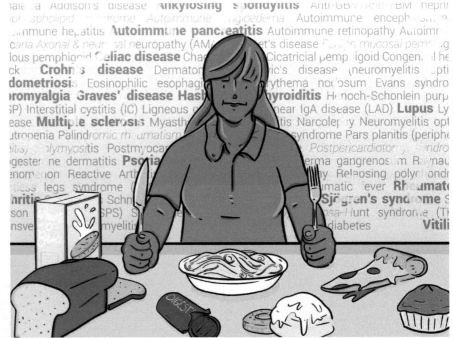

©2022 ALLIANCE FOR NATURAL HEALTH INTERNATIONAL

Too good to give up

The real problem is that most ultra-processed foods taste good - really good! Scarily, most have been designed to hit our 'bliss point', which essentially means that you gain maximum pleasure from eating them but are left wanting more and more and more. Eating them distorts the complex leptin/ghrelin regulation system that is central to our ability to properly regulate energy intake, satiety and hunger. We end up full of food, but we stay hungry and want to eat more. We're seduced by the ease of use and choice among what's on offer – plus they're available on every street corner, literally.

Given the stress in our lives, many of us also believe we should be able to treat ourselves.

As kids, we've accepted that we were always rewarded with foods that were intrinsically bad for us. As adults, the habit continues. We often know that such foods are bad for us, but we can't, won't or even flatly refuse to give them up. Recent research has highlighted that the high levels of ultra-processed foods bought by European households — and in the US — account for more than half of all calories consumed!

So, in the face of all the evidence pointing at their grave negative effects, how do these foods keep slipping into our shopping trolleys?

A smoking gun!

The tobacco industry did it, the food industry continues to do it with great success! Addiction is part of it – and distorting or ignoring the emerging science is another big part of it. It's surprising how much can be brushed under the carpet when you've bought the loyalty of scientists and public health organisations to help influence government guidelines. Far from being independently scientifically based, 'healthy eating' guidelines are just as much a political statement of the power and influence of the food industry.

Big Food's hold is alarming, often not acknowledged in political high places and is certainly not recognised by the average consumer. Powerful industry lobbies easily pull well-meaning advisory panel recommendations to pieces as the various players jockey for position to blunt and manipulate the language used in dietary guidelines, all in an effort to retain market share.

In the meantime, slick and well-orchestrated marketing campaigns often target children for their ability to influence parental purchasing decisions. Just think of the bombardment of mascot-led breakfast cereal commercials from a few years back, now thankfully a little more subdued. That vein of marketing has significantly changed our values. It's shaped us to assume if we get a takeaway or ready-meal it will save us time, stop arguments, keep everyone happy and that it's cheaper overall. As chronic disease levels rise, we're told to eat low fat, low sugar or even just smaller versions of the very foods causing the problem in the first place.

Cooking - optional

Sadly, families rarely eat together today. In the UK, only 1 in 5 people cook from scratch on a regular basis. Additionally, in the US, just 10% of people professed to even like cooking. Time spent in the kitchen is no longer necessary to feed ourselves and we're quickly losing the skills required to prepare food from scratch at home. Who has the few minutes to spare when we can easily whip out an app to order a takeaway or choose a meal from the plethora of ready-to-eat supermarket foods now available? Going out to eat is no longer an occasional treat, but the growing norm (or it was before the challenges of 2020!).

We hear that it's cheaper to buy processed foods at the supermarket rather than buying fresh food to cook at home. But this has not been our experience time and time again. It's definitely possible to buy whole foods that work out significantly cheaper than supermarket ready-made or take-away meals – but it's unfortunate that cooking is a dying art and not a skill children are learning in 'food technology' lessons at their schools.

Are those one-off, simple meals really as cheap or as nutritious as we think though? What's the true cost of the mass production of cheap ultra-processed foods? Economies of scale may mean the price we pay for an individual food item is low, but it doesn't take into account the use of energy, resources, impact of cheap labour and branching environmental damage. For those who like to shop ethically, there's a much larger impact at play behind the scenes, despite the cheery, enthusiastic packaging slapped on top.

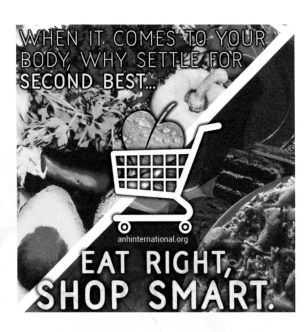

©2022 ALLIANCE FOR NATURAL HEALTH INTERNATIONAL

Take-out?
Take home!

It's never too late to learn to cook or prepare foods from scratch while experiencing the incredible effects of wholesome foods – as nature intended – on improving health, wellbeing and resilience. Even more important is the need to teach our children that reducing their reliance on ultra-processed and ready meals will improve their future health. Not only is it nowhere near as daunting or intimidating a task as some people think, cooking can actually be an incredibly fun and great way to bring social groups and families together. As the old adage says, teach someone to fish and you feed them for a lifetime! Parents lead by example, but there's plenty that can be done at school.

Oddly, in the UK, secondary schools' 'food technology' is still categorised under Design and Technology, which emphasises the technological aspects of cooking, rather than the biological and nutritional aspects of food. It would surely be far better to think of 'food science' as a subset of biology, given its role in nutrition. Such gaps in educating children on the importance of home cooking in opposition to processed food indulgence not only extenuates a culture of bad eating, it starves them of one of humankind's most essential and ancient skills!

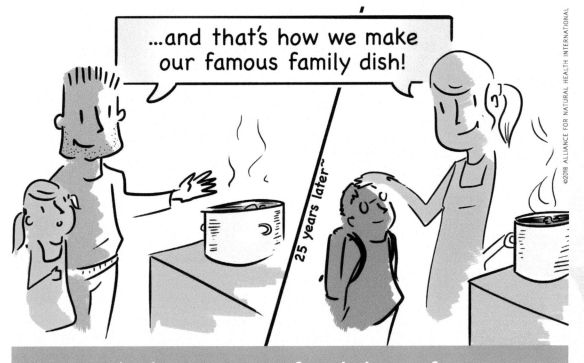

©2018 ALLIANCE FOR NATURAL HEALTH INTERNATIONAL

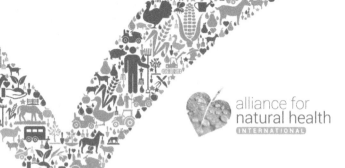

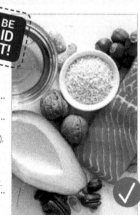

TOP 10 TIPS TO HELP YOU
EAT YOUR WAY TO BETTER HEALTH

1
EAT A RAINBOW EVERYDAY

- Consume vegetables and fruit that contain each of the **6 colours** of the phytonutrient spectrum (green, orange, red, yellow, blue/black/purple & white/tan).

- Pick up your handy 'Food and You' guide. Further info at www.**anhinternational.org/food4health**

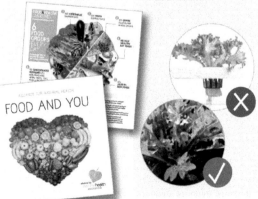

2
SOIL GROWN VEGETABLES ARE BEST

- Make sure your plant foods are grown in **rich, living soil.**

- Much of the supermarket salad veg today is grown in **glasshouse aquaponic systems** without soil.

- If your salad veg tastes watery, it's likely **deficient in lots of nutrients!**

3
BUY LOCAL/REGIONAL AND SEASONAL

- Try not to rely only on supermarket produce, most of which comes from **factory farms** and industrial-scale agriculture, and often from distant lands.

- Buy from the **'farm gate'**, from farmers' markets or have your organic produce delivered to your door via a **'box scheme'**.

- Buy food that's in season and when you do shop in supermarkets, make sure that most of your trolley has come from the living, fresh aisles and is **bar code free**.

- Ensure that processed foods and ready meals make up less than **15% of your diet.** Shopping can still be convenient, quick and cheap!

4
AVOID HIGHLY REFINED CARBS

- Cut out or **minimise sugar**, white bread, pastries, cakes, biscuits, pizza and white pasta.

- Replace these foods with more vegetables that are rich in complex, (rather than simple) carbs and fibre.

- Swap out fries and white potatoes for sweet potatoes or other root veg.

- Make sure that your meals and snacks include **good quality protein,** healthy fats, nuts, seeds and veg.

5

DON'T BE AFRAID OF FAT!

101 ON HEALTHY FAT SELECTION

- Fat doesn't make you fat!

- **Healthy fats** like avocados, coconut oil, nuts (not peanuts), extra virgin olive oil, oily fish, grass-fed beef, butter & ghee (unless intolerant) and eggs should be regulars in your diet.

- Other healthy plant oils include flax and hemp oils.

©2022 ALLIANCE FOR NATURAL HEALTH INTERNATIONAL

6

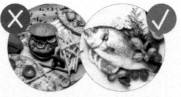

BALANCE YOUR OMEGA FATS

- We need **the right balance** of essential fatty acids (EFAs) for good health.

- Omega 3 fats (e.g. from oily fish) are necessary for our brains, eyes, nervous system and **every cell in the body**.

- Go easy on Omega 6 fats, which are particularly high in vegetable oils, seeds and processed foods. Replace with mono-unsaturated fats like olive oil.

- We've evolved to function on a ratio of Omega 6 to Omega 3 fats of around 3:1.

- Our modern, Western diets are typically more like 20:1 and are a major cause of persistent inflammation in our bodies, **a condition that underlies most chronic diseases.**

7

ANIMAL WELFARE STANDARDS

AVOID ANIMAL FOODS FROM FACTORY FARMS

Choose animal products from farming systems with **approved animal welfare standards**, and ones that don't use genetically modified animal feeds (cereals, soya, etc).

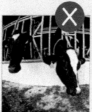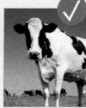

ABOUT US

Alliance for Natural Health International is an internationally-active, non-governmental organisation promoting natural and sustainable approaches to healthcare worldwide. Our catchcry is 'love nature, live naturally'.

ANH-Intl campaigns across a wide range of fields, including for freedom of choice in healthcare, healthy eating & lifestyles, and the use of micronutrients and herbal products in the management of our health and resilience. We operate campaigns that include drawing attention to misinformed, Big Food-influenced government healthy eating advice, to the uncertain science and risks of genetically modified foods, to the need for informed choice on vaccination and that aim to end mass fluoridation of drinking water supplies. We accomplish our mission through a unique application of 'good science' and 'good law'.

ANH-Intl was founded in 2002 by Robert Verkerk PhD, an internationally acclaimed expert in agricultural and health sustainability. Our international office is based in Dorking, UK, while our US base (www.anh-usa.org) operates out of Atlanta, Georgia.

8

AVOID HIGHLY PROCESSED, 'WHOLE GRAIN' CEREALS

- These cereals are highly mechanically processed and spike blood glucose **just like sugary, refined cereals.**

- They don't make you feel full.

- They burn fast, contributing to mid-morning lows and make you want to eat more!

- Many are also **high in sugar** before adding sugar or honey like so many people do.

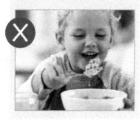

9

AS MUCH AS 30g SUGAR IN A 330ml CAN OF FIZZY DRINK

BEVERAGES: THE GOOD, BAD AND THE UGLY

- **Eat your calories, don't drink them!**

- Fizzy drinks and fruit juices can be a hideous source of hidden sugars.

- Check labels before drinking and **avoid artificial sweeteners.**

- **Drink alcohol in moderation** – red wine contains resveratrol which has many beneficial properties!

- Tea and coffee are dehydrating not hydrating – **your body is 70% water.**

- Fresh spring or filtered water is what your body really needs - **your body will thank you for 1.5 litres per day**, more if you're exercising or the weather's hot.

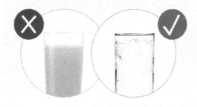

10

FOOD PREP AND COOKING GUIDELINES

- Avoid prolonged high temperature cooking like **frying and grilling**.

- Briefly searing meat or fish to seal in the goodness is advised.

- Proteins, fats and vegetables are very sensitive to **heat damage**.

- **Treat your food kindly** with lower temperature cooking.

- Minimise charred or toasted foods which contain **cancer-causing** chemicals.

- Get experimenting with a slow cooker!

PLEASE HELP US SPREAD THE WORD

Information is power. Please help others to benefit from this information and that's where your help is vital. ANH-Intl is a non-profit organisation that survives on donations from people like you. So please help us today by making a donation.

Donations can be made securely via www.anhinternational.org/donate

www.anhinternational.org

anhinternational
anhcampaign
ANHIntl

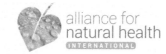
alliance for natural health INTERNATIONAL

©2022 ALLIANCE FOR NATURAL HEALTH INTERNATIONAL

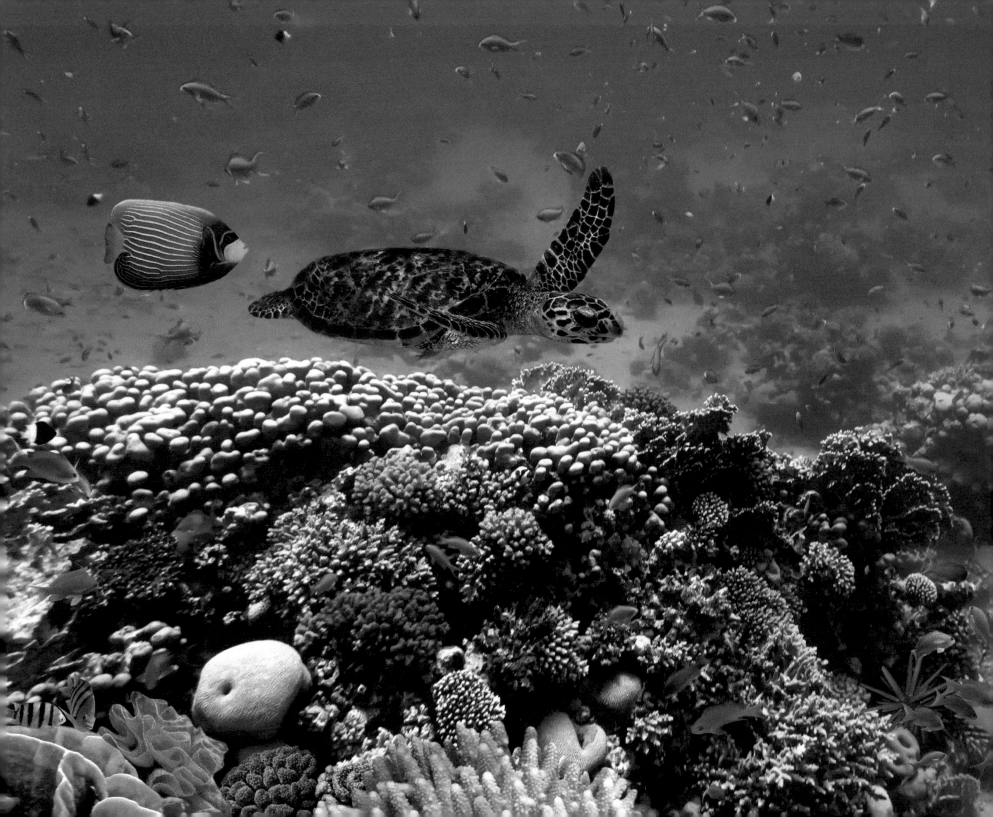

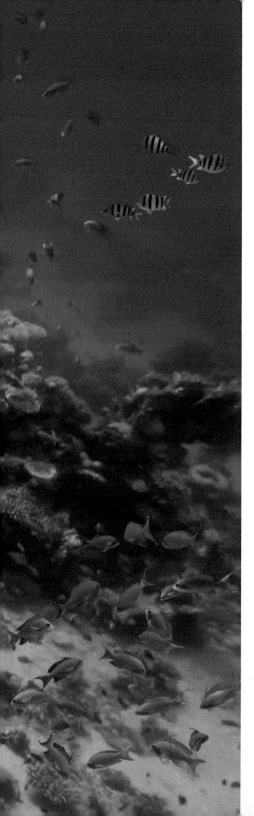

The human dietary diversity crisis

Earth's biodiversity is in decline. Be it animals or plants, or the microorganisms in our agricultural soils or guts, the number of species at risk of extinction as a result of human activity grows every day. Globalisation and industrialisation have had other untoward effects as well. One of these is the dramatic change not only in the types of food available to us, but also in the diversity of nutrients found in those foods. Today's plant foods come with a very different nutrient profile compared with those of our paleolithic ancestors. The same can be said of the farm animals on which many humans continue to rely as a major component of their protein intake. All of this, while we continue to carry genes that have barely changed from those of our Paleolithic ancestors, must have consequences.

The consequences of what is referred to scientifically as 'dietary simplification' are enormous. So much so that it likely underpins a significant part of the chronic disease crisis we see today and may well be part of your health picture too.

Why does diversity matter?

Our entire planet has evolved using diversity to stay healthy and in balance. Just look at the diversity in a rainforest or a coral reef and you'll understand that our bodies, and our environment, are mirror images. We need layers of diversity to maintain stability within living systems, to stop one species taking over to the detriment of another, be they human, animal, plant or microbial.

HUMAN DIETARY DIVERSITY CRISIS

SINCE THE 1900'S...

Ref 1

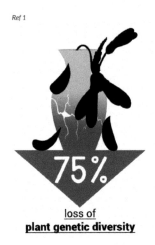

75%

loss of
plant genetic diversity

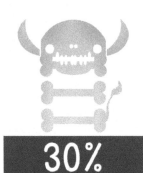

30%

livestock breeds at
risk of extinction

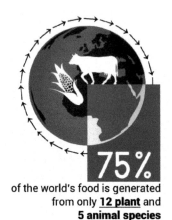

75%

of the world's food is generated
from only **12 plant** and
5 animal species

Ref 2

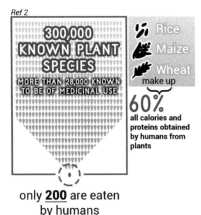

300,000 KNOWN PLANT SPECIES

MORE THAN 28,000 KNOWN TO BE OF MEDICINAL USE

only **200** are eaten
by humans

Rice
Maize
Wheat
make up

60%
all calories and
proteins obtained
by humans from
plants

Ref 3

REDUCTIONS IN NUTRIENTS BETWEEN 1940-1991	
Vegetables	Fruit
Calcium (Ca) –46%	Sodium (Na) – 29%
Magnesium (Mg) –24%	Magnesium (Mg) –16%
Copper (Cu) –76%	Iron (Fe) –24%
Sodium (Na) –49%	Copper (Cu) –20%
Potassium (K) –16%	Potassium (K) –19%
Iron (Fe) –27%	Phosphorus (P) +2%
Phosphorus (P) +9%	Calcium (Ca) –16%
	Zinc (Zn) –27%

OH, HOW THE TIMES HAVE CHANGED!

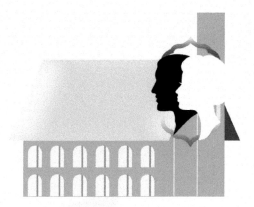

Ref 4

3,000 to 4,500 calories per day (men) and 2,750 to 3,500 (women) mid Victorians, high levels of physical exercise (Mid-Victorian working class men and women consumed between 50% and 100% more calories than we do)

All fruits and vegetables were organically grown, and therefore had higher levels of phytonutrients than the intensively grown crops we eat today

Consumption of fruits and vegetables amounting to 8 to 10 portions per day - today's average at 3.5 portions per day

Victorian diet also contained significantly more nuts, legumes, whole grains and omega three fatty acids than the modern diet

Increased consumption of offal, which has a higher micronutrient density than the skeletal muscle we largely eat today. Plus all important nucleotides, the building blocks of DNA

Ref 5

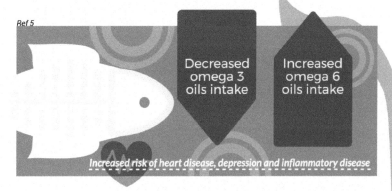

Decreased omega 3 oils intake

Increased omega 6 oils intake

Increased risk of heart disease, depression and inflammatory disease

Ref 6

Diets high in vegetables & fruit have been associated with reduced cancer risk

It's particularly the bitter phytochemicals that are cancer-protective. Debittering of foods to make them more acceptable to consumers is bad for health

Ref 7, 8, 9

ORGANIC MEAT AND MILK

60% higher levels of antioxidants

⬆ **Omega 3 fatty acids, myristic and palmitic acid**

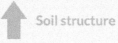

40% more CLA conjugated linoleic acid

⬆ **Fat soluble vitamins vitamin E and carotenoids (vitamin A)**

Ref 10

Recommended ratio of omega 6:omega 3 is 3:1

Average ratio found in grass fed beef	Average ratio found in grain fed beef
1.53:1	**7.65:1**

Ref 11

Organic Strawberries

8.5%	more antioxidants
9.7%	more ascorbic acid
10.5%	more phenolics

Organic Soil

21.6%	more carbon
30.2%	more nitrogen
159.4%	more microbial biomass

⬆ Soil structure

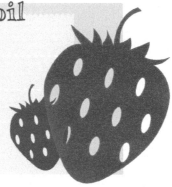

Ref 12

And it's not just food. Diverse phytonutrients in food-based supplements can reduce inflammation, epigenetically alter gene expression, at the root.

✓

Ref 13

THE MORE VEGETABLES AND FRUIT, THE MORE BACTERIAL DIVERSITY!

Love your bugs and they'll love you back!

Our microbes are our partners in health, we can't be healthy and happy without them being healthy and happy...

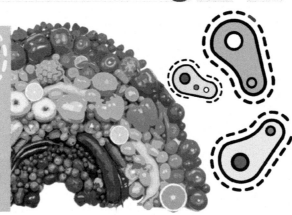

IT'S ALL ABOUT THE SUM OF THE PARTS!

Ref 14, 15.

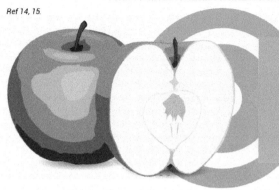

Whole fruit = synergistic antioxidant and anticancer effects (the different phytochemicals in plants work together and compliment each other, enhancing their effects)

Microbes are part of the ecosystem within our bodies that we've evolved with. They are integral to our health. Fewer microbes and poor diversity directly translates to poorer health.

Ref 16

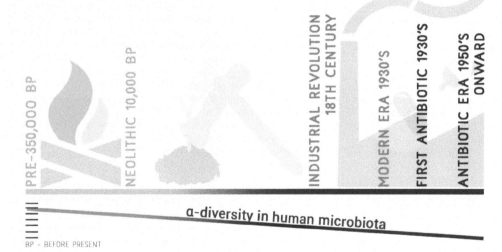

PRE-350,000 BP

NEOLITHIC 10,000 BP

INDUSTRIAL REVOLUTION 18TH CENTURY

MODERN ERA 1930'S

FIRST ANTIBIOTIC 1930'S

ANTIBIOTIC ERA 1950'S ONWARD

α-diversity in human microbiota

BP - BEFORE PRESENT

References:
anhinternational.org/wp-content/uploads/2017/06/170628-Diversity-References-1.pdf

anhinternational.org
©2017 Alliance for Natural Health International

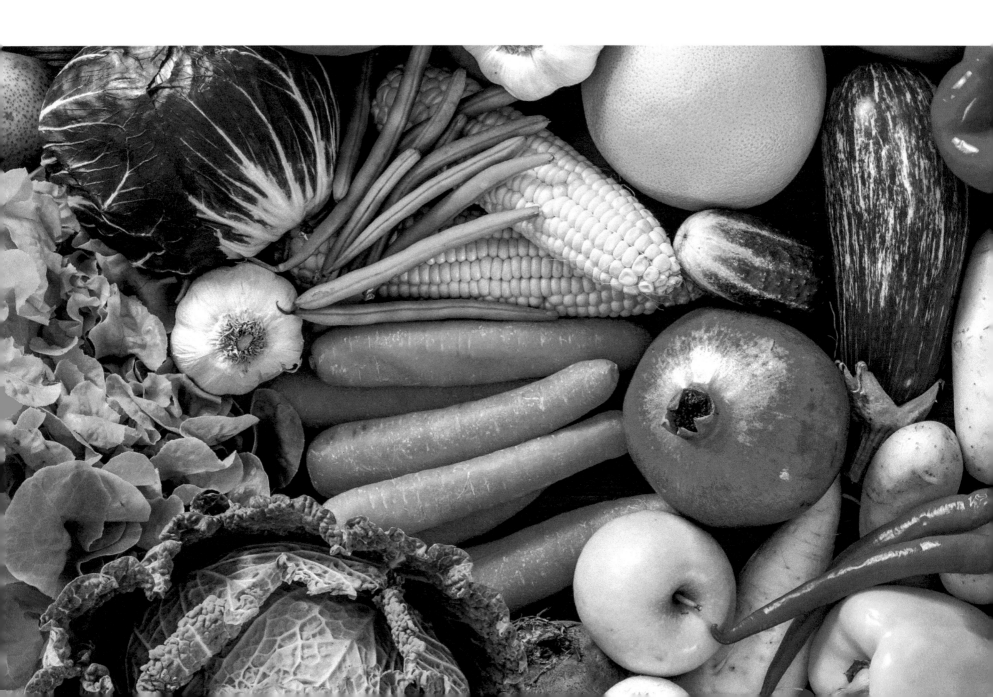

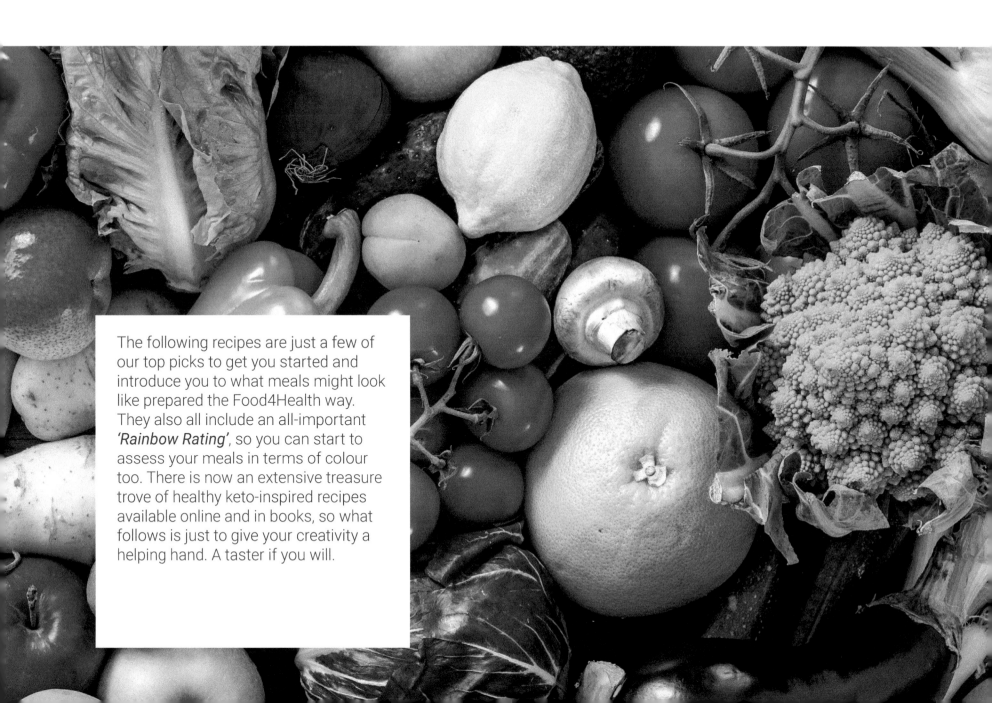

EATING THE FOOD4HEALTH WAY:
A FEW KICKSTARTER RECIPES

The following recipes are just a few of our top picks to get you started and introduce you to what meals might look like prepared the Food4Health way. They also all include an all-important *'Rainbow Rating'*, so you can start to assess your meals in terms of colour too. There is now an extensive treasure trove of healthy keto-inspired recipes available online and in books, so what follows is just to give your creativity a helping hand. A taster if you will.

BREAKFAST

COCONUT PANCAKES

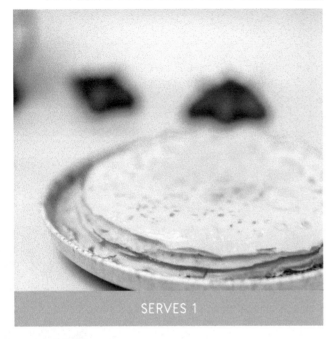

SERVES 1

INGREDIENTS:

- 2 eggs
- 1tbsp Coconut flour
- Coconut oil for cooking

METHOD:

1. Beat the eggs
2. Add the coconut flour and mix thoroughly (the coconut flour may form lumps, but the mixture will cook properly)
3. Heat the coconut oil in a pan (medium heat) and add the egg mixture, either in two separate 'pancakes' or one large 'pancake'. Cook until browned on the first side, turn over and cook the second side
4. Serve with coconut cream, mixed nuts or seeds, a drizzle of maple syrup (if desired), sliced banana, berries or stewed apple.

©2022 ALLIANCE FOR NATURAL HEALTH INTERNATIONAL

EGG MUFFINS

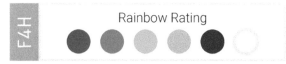

Rainbow Rating

INGREDIENTS:

12 eggs (one per muffin) beaten

Optional filling ideas (pick 2 or 3)

- 50 g grated cheese
- 12 baby tomatoes chopped (1 per muffin)
- ½ medium courgette, grated
- 1 small carrot, grated
- 50 g peas
- 50 g sweetcorn
- 4 finely chopped spring onions
- ½ finely chopped bell pepper
- 4 small finely chopped mushrooms

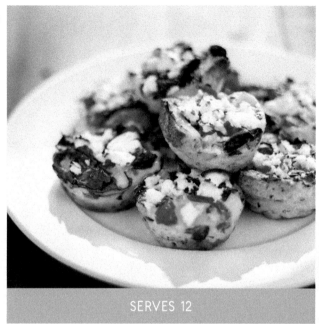

SERVES 12

METHOD:

1. Preheat oven to 180°C/350°F
2. Grease a 12 hole muffin tin or line with baking paper
3. Beat the eggs
4. Divide your desired fillings between each muffin cup
5. Top up with beaten egg (each cup holds 1 egg)
6. Cook for 15-20 mins until golden.

These freeze really well so can be made in advance and taken out when needed. Because they are individual everyone can choose their preferred fillings.

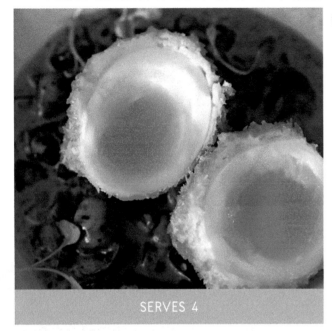

SERVES 4

MUSHROOM RAGOUT WITH POACHED EGGS

V

INGREDIENTS:

- 15 g dried porcini mushrooms
- 600 ml water
- 600 g mixed fresh mushrooms
- 100 ml olive oil
- 2 garlic cloves, crushed
- 1 medium onion diced
- 1 medium carrot, peeled and diced
- 3 celery sticks, cut into pieces

- 120 ml white wine (if tolerated) or vegetable stock with a tbsp of apple cider vinegar
- 100 g soured cream (if tolerated) or unsweetened coconut yogurt
- 1 tbsp thyme
- 4 tbsp mixed chopped fresh tarragon and parsley
- Pink Himalayan salt and black pepper
- 8 eggs (2 per person), poached

METHOD:

1. Soak the dried porcini mushrooms in 200 ml of the water for 30 minutes. While they soak clean your fresh mushrooms and cut them up into chunks
2. Preheat the oven to 200°C/400°F
3. Put a tablespoon of olive oil into a medium saucepan and cook the mushrooms in batches until they're lightly browned
4. Remove all the mushrooms from the pan and add the carrot, garlic, onion and celery into the pan with another tablespoon of olive oil. Cook over a medium heat for 5 minutes, then add the wine or stock and vinegar
5. Remove the porcini mushrooms from the soaking water, squeeze out any excess liquid and put to one side
6. Pour the soaking liquid through a strainer to remove any grit then add to the pan with the remaining water, thyme and season with salt and pepper. Simmer for 20 minutes, or until the liquid has reduced by half
7. While the stock is reducing, poach the eggs to your liking and place in iced water until needed
8. Once the stock has reduced, strain to remove the vegetables and return the stock to the pan. Add all the mushrooms, the cream or yogurt, chopped fresh herbs and salt and pepper to taste
9. Serve topped with 2 poached eggs per person.

©2022 ALLIANCE FOR NATURAL HEALTH INTERNATIONAL

OVERNIGHT KETO 'OATS'

F4H

Rainbow Rating

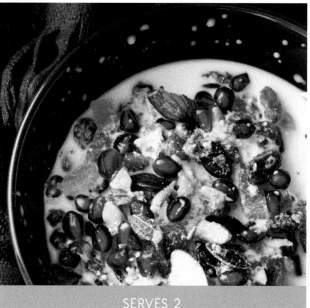

V

VE

SERVES 2

INGREDIENTS:

- 50 g almond butter
- 160 g coconut milk (full fat)
- 75 g hemp seed
- 20 g chia seeds
- 25 g pecans, roughly chopped
- 25 g almonds, roughly chopped
- 25 g walnuts, roughly chopped
- 15 g pumpkin seeds
- 15 g sunflower seeds

To top:

- 20 g berries of your choice
- 10 g desiccated coconut

METHOD:

1. Mix all the ingredients (except the berries and coconut) together in a bowl
2. Pop in the fridge and leave to soak overnight
3. Refresh with a little coconut milk in the morning if the consistency is too dense and serve topped with the berries and desiccated coconut.

VEGAN

Rainbow Rating

F4H

V

VE

SERVES 2 – 4

OVERNIGHT OATMEAL

INGREDIENTS:

- 1 cup of gluten-free rough, jumbo or steel cut porridge oats
- 2 scoops (25g) protein powder (avoid whey!) - optional
- A pinch of sea/Himalayan salt
- ½ tsp vanilla extract
- 2 tbsp organic, naturally derived coconut MCT oil
- 150 ml unsweetened almond or coconut milk (or other non-dairy milk of your choice)

- 150 ml unsweetened apple juice
- 1 tsp unsweetened cocoa powder
- 100 g chopped nuts – walnuts, pecans, macadamia or almonds work well, but any nuts will do

Optional toppings: desiccated coconut, grated apple, berries, a handful of seeds or a spoon of nut butter

METHOD:

1. In a small bowl, mix all of the ingredients together (except for toppings)
2. Divide the mixture between 4 bowls, mugs, or mason jars. You can divide in half for two large servings
3. Cover and refrigerate overnight (or for at least 2 hours) so the oats soften and absorb the liquid. *NB: You'll need to let them soak overnight if using steel cut oats*

4. Just before serving, add toppings and enjoy cold, or gently heat in a saucepan for a speedy winter warmer. If you're heating your oatmeal, then don't add the toppings until serving
5. Serve with some extra non-dairy milk or coconut yoghurt.

Cook's Tip: If you find your oatmeal a little dry after soaking, just top up with a little water and remix.

©2022 ALLIANCE FOR NATURAL HEALTH INTERNATIONAL

PROTEIN POWER SUPER SMOOTHIE

CAN BE MADE VEGAN

F4H

Rainbow Rating
● ○ ○ ○ ● ●

V

INGREDIENTS:

- ¼ cup milk (Organic, A2, Coconut, Oat or other plant-based milk of your choice)
- 1 banana (peeled and frozen)
- ½ cup raspberries
- ½ tbsp molasses
- ¼ tsp ginger powder

- ¼ tsp cinnamon
- 1 tbsp oats
- 1 tbsp shredded coconut
- 1 serving protein powder (avoid whey if dairy intolerant)

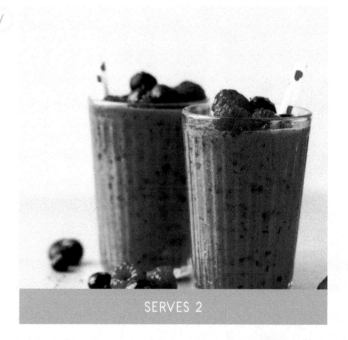

SERVES 2

METHOD:

Add ingredients to a blender and blend till smooth and creamy.

VEGAN

Rainbow Rating

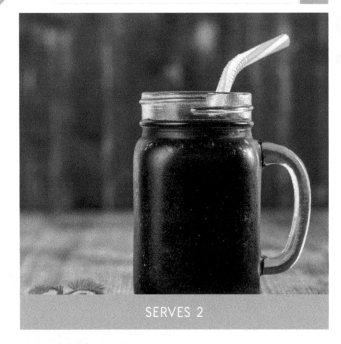

SERVES 2

RAINBOW VEG SMOOTHIE

INGREDIENTS:

- 250 ml water – more if required to reach desired consistency
- ½ cup / 75 g loosely washed and roughly chopped kale
- ½ cup / 75 g washed and roughly chopped spinach
- 1 small carrot
- 1 stick of celery
- 1 avocado
- 1 green apple, washed, cored and quartered but not peeled
- ½ raw beetroot
- 50 g raspberries
- 50 g blackberries / blueberries
- 2 cm root ginger (add more if you like ginger!)
- 2 tbsp milled flax seeds
- 1-2 limes, juiced (according to taste)
- 1-2 scoops of a whey-free protein powder (optional)

METHOD:

Add the water to a food processor, liquidiser, Vitamix or Nutribullet, then add the other ingredients and blend on high speed till thoroughly combined. Add more water, if necessary, to reach desired consistency.

©2022 ALLIANCE FOR NATURAL HEALTH INTERNATIONAL

THAI OMELETTE

Rainbow Rating

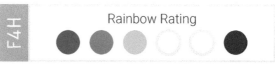

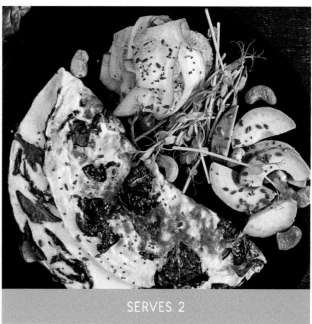

SERVES 2

INGREDIENTS:

- 6 large eggs
- Juice ½ lime
- 1 tbsp coconut oil
- 1 clove garlic, crushed
- 20 g fresh root ginger, grated
- 1 tbsp tamari
- 2 tsp sesame oil
- 30 g cashew nuts

- 100 g tempeh
- 1 bunch spring onions
- 1 pack coriander, chopped
- Himalayan pink salt and ground black pepper
- 1 large avocado, sliced
- Lime wedges

METHOD:

1. Beat the eggs with the lime juice and season with salt and pepper
2. Add half coconut oil to a frying pan and heat
3. Add the tempeh and cook until golden brown. Add the ginger and garlic and fry for a couple of mins. Remove the pan from the heat and stir through the chilli, tamari, cashew nuts and sesame oil. Tip into a bowl and put to one side
4. Clean the pan and add the rest of the coconut oil. Heat the oil. Add half the egg mixture to the pan and cook until browned on one side. Flip over and cook until browned. Place on a warm plate. Repeat for the second omelette
5. Top the omelettes with finely sliced spring onions, sliced avocado, chopped coriander and the chilli cashew nut and tempeh mixture with lime wedges on the side.

Cook's Tip: Serve with lightly steamed green beans and broccoli.

CAN BE MADE VEGAN

Rainbow Rating

F4H

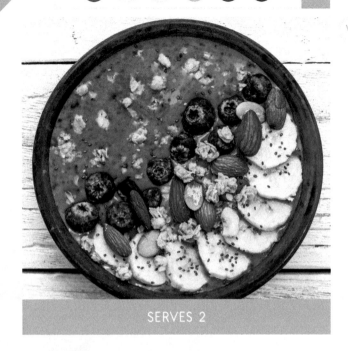

SERVES 2

WARM WINTER FRUIT BOWL

INGREDIENTS:

- 150 g frozen mixed berries
- 100 g raw mixed nuts (chopped) - optional
- 1 tsp chia seeds
- 1 tbsp coconut oil
- A pinch of nutmeg
- A pinch of ground cloves
- ½ tsp natural vanilla essence
- Warm milk (Organic, A2, Almond, Coconut or Oat)

- A dollop of coconut yoghurt or natural bio/live yoghurt (if not dairy intolerant)
- Sprinkle of sunflower and pumpkin seeds

Optional:
Drizzle of honey

METHOD:

1. Add the berry, nut and chia seed (or alternative) mix to an ovenproof dish
2. Add 2 tbsp water, 1 tbsp coconut oil, the vanilla essence and the spices. Mix well, cover and bake in a low oven (150°C/300°F) till hot (in a fan oven, this will take about 20 mins, but check at 15 mins)
3. Pour over warm milk and finish with a dollop of yoghurt, a drizzle of honey and a sprinkle of seeds.

Note: If you cut out the nuts, to increase the protein level you can also add some soaked quinoa to the mix.

©2022 ALLIANCE FOR NATURAL HEALTH INTERNATIONAL

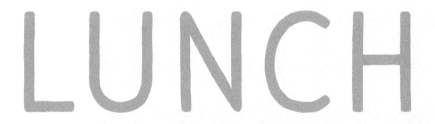

KICKSTARTER RECIPES:

LUNCH

Rainbow Rating

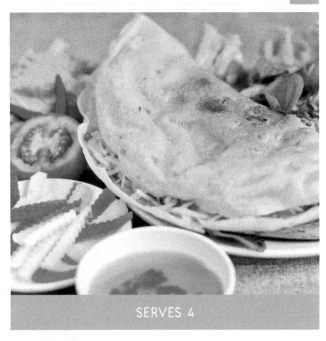

SERVES 4

BANH XEO – SAVOURY PANCAKES WITH NUTS AND PRAWNS

INGREDIENTS:

Pancakes

- 200 g rice flour
- 2 eggs - or equivalent egg replacer
- ½ tsp salt
- 1 tsp ground turmeric
- 400 ml canned coconut milk (full fat)
- Coconut or olive oil for frying

Sauce

- 40 ml lime juice
- 1 ½ tbsp toasted sesame oil
- 1 tbsp brown sugar
- 1 tbsp rice wine vinegar or apple cider vinegar
- 1 tbsp tamari
- 2 tbsp grated fresh root ginger
- 1 fresh red chilli finely chopped (to your taste)
- 1 clove garlic, crushed
- ½ tsp Himalayan pink salt

Filling

- 300 g cooked king prawns
- 1 large carrot cut into matchsticks
- 150 g flaked almonds or finely chopped cashews
- 30 g pack radishes cut into matchsticks
- 4 spring onions
- 1 fresh green chilli finely sliced
- 80 g mangetout lightly steamed
- 15 g coriander
- 15 g Thai basil (or standard basil)
- 15 g mint
- 100 g mung bean sprouts
- 100 g enoki mushrooms (optional)

©2022 ALLIANCE FOR NATURAL HEALTH INTERNATIONAL

METHOD:

1. Make the batter by putting the flour, egg, salt and turmeric in a large bowl and mixing together. Slowly add the coconut milk, whisking well to avoid lumps. The batter should be the consistency of single cream. If it's too thick add a little water to thin it out. Put to one side to rest
2. Make the sauce by whisking all the ingredients together
3. Prepare the vegetables and nuts
4. Heat a non-stick frying pan and add olive or coconut oil to the pan
5. Add a ladle full of batter to the pan, swirl round and cook until the underside is golden. Turn the pancake over to cook the other side. Pop on a plate resting in a low oven (100°C/200°F) while you cook the rest of the pancakes. This mixture will make 4 large pancakes or 6-8 smaller pancakes
6. Mix the vegetables, prawns and nuts together in the sauce so they're well coated
7. Put a pancake on a plate, pile with the veggies and sauce, fold into a spring roll shape and enjoy.

Cook's Tip: If you can't eat nuts, then substitute with tempeh or legumes to keep your protein levels up.

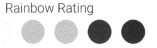

VEGAN

Rainbow Rating

F4H

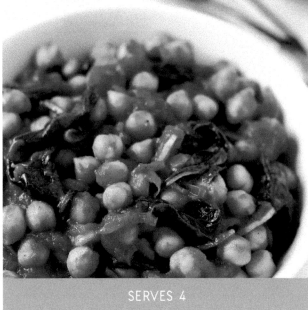

SERVES 4

V

VE

CHICKPEAS WITH SEA SALAD AND STAR ANISE

INGREDIENTS:

- 2 tbsp olive oil, ghee or coconut oil
- 1 tbsp mustard seeds
- 1 tsp fennel seeds
- ½ tsp nigella seeds
- 8 cloves garlic finely chopped
- 1 tbsp grated fresh root ginger
- 200 g tomato puree
- 2-4 green chillies finely chopped (to your taste)
- ½ tsp ground turmeric or 1 tsp grated fresh turmeric

- ½ tsp chilli powder
- 6 star anise
- 1 tsp ground ginger
- 1 tsp Himalayan salt
- 2 tbsp sea salad (available from health food shops)
- 2 x 400 g can chickpeas, rinsed and drained
- Chopped fresh coriander to garnish

METHOD:

1. Add the mustard, fennel and nigella seeds to a dry pan and gently heat, moving them around so they don't burn. As soon as you start to smell the spice aroma, add the ghee or oil and cook over a medium heat until they start to pop (1-2 minutes)

2. Add the garlic and cook until it starts to sizzle. Add the fresh ginger and chillies and cook until the ginger starts to brown (keep stirring). Add the turmeric and chilli powder and cook for a further 20 seconds

3. Add the tomato puree, mix well and heat through then add the star anise, ground ginger, salt and sea salad. Add 750 ml boiling water and bring to a simmer. Add the chickpeas and simmer uncovered for 20 minutes

4. Garnish with the chopped coriander before serving.

©2022 ALLIANCE FOR NATURAL HEALTH INTERNATIONAL

CREAMY VEGETABLE SOUP

Rainbow Rating

VEGAN

V

VE

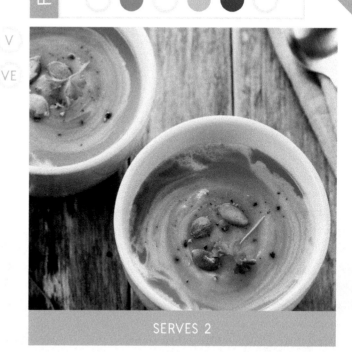

SERVES 2

INGREDIENTS:

- 1 leek sliced
- 1 onion diced
- 1 clove garlic
- 1 medium carrot diced
- 100 g broccoli
- 100 g selection of green leafy veg e.g. watercress, spinach, kale

- 4 heaped tablespoons humous
- 2 tbsp chopped fresh tarragon
- 1 L vegetable stock

METHOD:

1. Fry the leek, onion and garlic gently until soft
2. Add the carrot, broccoli, tarragon and veg stock
3. Bring to the boil and simmer until the veg is nearly cooked
4. Add the green leafy veg and simmer for another 5 minutes
5. Put the soup into a blender and blend
6. Add the humous
7. Pulse to combine.

Season to taste and serve with a swirl of olive oil, natural, live, yoghurt (if tolerated) or dairy-free alternative.

Rainbow Rating

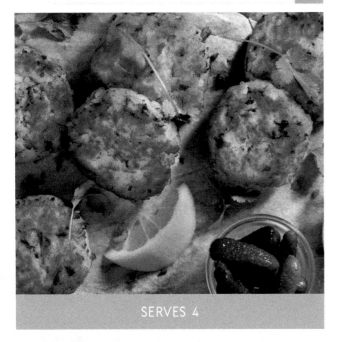

SERVES 4

EASY SALMON FISHCAKES

INGREDIENTS:

- 4 salmon fillets, skinned
- 5 cm piece of ginger, peeled and grated
- 1 clove of garlic, crushed
- Zest of a lime (or lemon)
- Squeeze of lime juice (or lemon)
- Coconut or olive oil for frying
- Salt and pepper to taste
- 2 tbsp chopped fresh parsley or 1 tbsp chopped Thai basil for a more eastern flavour

METHOD:

1. Put the first 7 ingredients into a food processor and blend to a paste
2. Transfer to a mixing bowl and add in the fresh herbs
3. Form into palm sized patties (makes approx 9)
4. Fry in a little coconut or olive oil until cooked through
5. Serve with green veg and a large mixed salad.

Cook's Tip: For a more Asian flavour with a bit of heat, spice up your patties with half a tsp of Sambal Oelek.

©2022 ALLIANCE FOR NATURAL HEALTH INTERNATIONAL

EGG BAKED AVOCADO

Rainbow Rating

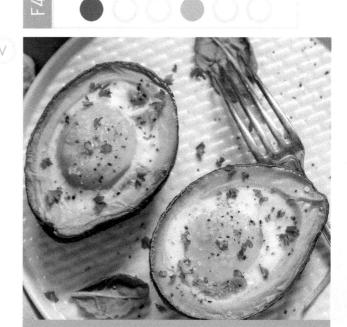

SERVES 4

INGREDIENTS:

- 2 large ripe avocados, halved and pitted
- 4 large eggs
- ¼ red onion or 1 shallot or 2 spring onions
- 1 tsp paprika
- 1 lime or ½ lemon
- Himalayan pink salt and ground black pepper
- Freshly chopped chives, for garnish

METHOD:

1. Preheat oven to 180°C/350°F. Scoop about 1 tablespoon worth of avocado out of each half and reserve in the fridge with a little lemon or lime juice squeezed across the top

2. Place hollowed avocados in a baking dish, then crack eggs into a bowl, one at a time. Using a spoon, transfer one yolk to each avocado half, then spoon in as much egg white as you can fit without spilling over

3. Season with salt and pepper and bake until whites are set and yolks are no longer runny - 20 to 25 minutes (cover with foil if avocados are beginning to brown)

4. Whilst the avocados are baking, make a side garnish from the reserved avocado by mixing it with finely chopped red onion (shallots or spring onions will work too), paprika and salt and pepper to taste. You will already have squeezed some lime or lemon over it, but add more to taste.

Cook's Tip: Serve with vegan 'bacon' or the real thing if you're an omnivore!

Rainbow Rating

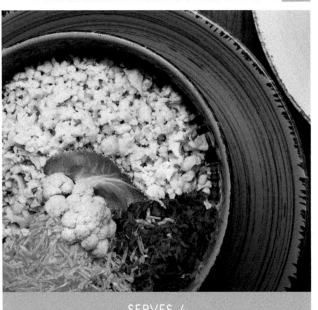

SERVES 4

EGG FRIED VEGGIE RICE

INGREDIENTS:

- ½ head cauliflower, broken into florets
- 1 head broccoli, broken into florets
- 2 medium carrots, peeled and chopped into pieces
- 1 medium raw beetroot, peeled and diced
- 1 small courgette, grated (yellow if available)
- Olive oil or coconut oil
- 3 cloves garlic, crushed
- 1 medium onion, diced
- 1 medium bell pepper, diced

- 1 tbsp minced fresh ginger
- 1 tbsp fresh turmeric, grated
- 4-5 tbsp tamari
- Chopped chilli to taste (optional)
- 75 g ea frozen peas / green beans
- 1 bunch parsley
- 4 eggs
- Sea salt and ground black pepper

METHOD:

1. Take frozen peas and beans out of the freezer and leave to defrost
2. Beat the eggs in a bowl
3. Prepare the veg rice by blitzing the cauliflower, broccoli, carrots and beetroot (one at a time) in a food processor until they resemble rice or chop finely
4. Mix the veg rice in a large bowl
5. Heat 1 tbsp oil in a large, non-stick frying pan or wok. If using bacon, add and fry until cooked through. Remove from pan and put on a plate

6. Add the onion and pepper and cook for 5 mins until slightly softened. Add the ginger, garlic and spices. Cook briefly to release the oils from the spices
7. Add the riced vegetables and Tamari to the pan and stir everything together. Add the green beans and peas, and cook, stirring, for 1-2 mins until heated through. Push the veg mix to one side of the pan. Add the eggs and scramble. Mix the scrambled egg though the vegetable mix

8. Season with salt and pepper to taste
9. Sprinkle with desired toppings and serve.

Toppings:

- *For omnivores: leftover roast chicken, prawns or bacon (optional)*
- *1 bunch spring onions (scallions) sliced*
- *Chopped avocado*
- *Sweetcorn*

©2022 ALLIANCE FOR NATURAL HEALTH INTERNATIONAL

GREEN TORTILLA

F4H

Rainbow Rating

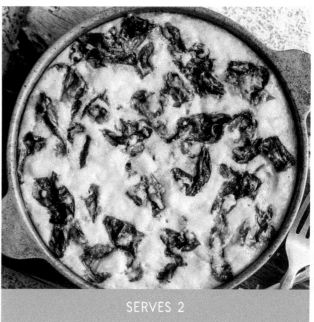

SERVES 2

INGREDIENTS:

- 6 large eggs
- 1 tbsp olive oil
- 1 small (or half a medium red) onion finely chopped
- 1 clove garlic, crushed
- 1 tsp basil (fresh or dried)
- 1 tsp oregano (fresh or dried)
- Handful parsley chopped

- 100 g spinach or kale sliced
- 50 g fennel chopped into small pieces
- 100 g peas
- Himalayan pink salt and ground black pepper

METHOD:

1. Heat half the olive oil in a frying pan. Add the onion and cook until soft. Add the garlic and herbs along with the spinach, peas and fennel and a little water. Cook for 3-5 minutes until just soft
2. Beat the eggs with the herbs and vegetables then season with salt and pepper
3. Turn on the grill to a medium heat
4. Heat the rest of the oil in the pan, then add the egg mixture

5. Turn the heat down and cook for approx. 5 minutes until the mixture starts to set and is coming away from the sides of the pan
6. Put the pan under the grill to cook the top and middle.

Cook's Tip: Serve with sliced tomatoes and mozzarella, scattered with more basil.

CAN BE MADE VEGAN

Rainbow Rating

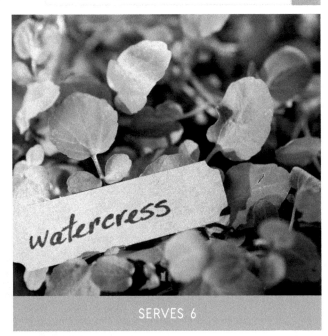

watercress

SERVES 6

LONGEVITY WATERCRESS SOUP

INGREDIENTS:

- 1.5 litres of rich bone broth or vegetable stock
- Fresh lemon or lime juice (2 tbsp)
- Gluten-free tamari (Japanese soya sauce)

- 1 packet (approx 100g) watercress
- 4 eggs
- Salt and pepper to taste
- Fresh coriander (optional)
- 2 tbsp sesame seeds

METHOD:

1. Gently warm the bone broth or vegetable stock to near boiling and add tamari, lemon/lime juice, salt and pepper to taste
2. Toast the sesame seeds in a dry frying pan, turning them over regularly and being careful not to burn them. As soon as they're toasted remove them to a plate so they don't cook any further
3. Separate the egg whites, set the yolks aside and beat the raw egg whites with a fork

4. Pour into the hot broth, beating gently with a fork until stringy
5. Just before serving, place the washed, chopped (approx 2.5 cm lengths) watercress, including leaves and stalks (discard any woody ones) into the broth
6. Add coarsely chopped coriander (1 tbsp per bowl)
7. Sprinkle the broth with toasted sesame seeds and serve.

©2022 ALLIANCE FOR NATURAL HEALTH INTERNATIONAL

NUTTY SEEDY BREAD

Rainbow Rating

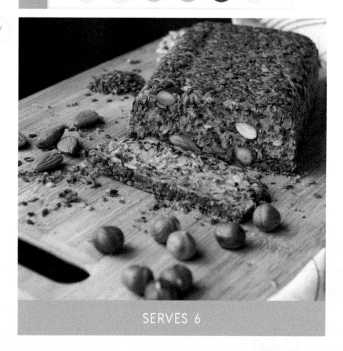

SERVES 6

INGREDIENTS:

- 100 g almonds
- 100 g walnuts
- 100 g sunflower seeds
- 100 g pumpkin seeds
- 100 g linseeds
- 100 g sesame seeds
- 5 eggs
- 100 ml olive oil
- 100 ml water
- Pinch of salt

Great with soup or as a breakfast with nut butter.

METHOD:

1. Preheat the oven to 160°C/320°F
2. Put everything in a bowl and mix (or in your blender if you'd rather have a smoother texture)
3. Grease a 1 litre loaf tin with coconut oil and line with baking paper
4. Pour the mixture into the tin and bake for 1 hour
5. Turn out and allow to cool a little before slicing.

With thanks to our friend Karina Athwal for sharing this one.

CAN BE MADE VEGAN

Rainbow Rating

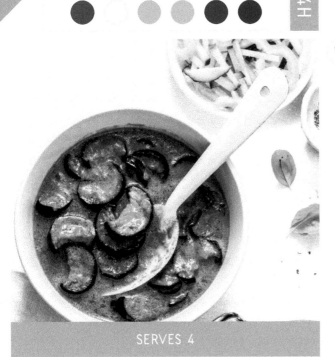

SERVES 4

F4H

V

OVEN ROASTED AUBERGINE AND TOMATOES IN YOGURT SAUCE

INGREDIENTS:

- 2 tbsp olive oil
- 2 tsp cumin seeds
- 1 tsp ground coriander
- ¾ tsp sea or pink Himalayan salt
- 1 small onion sliced
- 4 cloves garlic crushed
- 2-4 green chillies, finely chopped (depending on preference, optional)
- 3 large aubergines, or 900 g baby aubergines
- 4 large fresh tomatoes

- 1 tsp turmeric
- 1 tbsp tomato purée
- 4 tbsp full fat Greek yogurt (dairy or non-dairy)
- 1 lime

METHOD:

1. Preheat the oven to 200°C/fan 180°C/400°F
2. Prick the aubergines with a fork then place the whole aubergines and the tomatoes on a baking tray. Bake in the oven for approx 25 minutes or until soft to the touch
3. Pour the olive oil into a deep saucepan and heat over a medium heat. Add the cumin seeds and cook until they start to pop (2-3 minutes). Add the salt and onion and fry until the onion is light brown, stirring frequently (approx. 5 minutes)

4. Add the garlic and chilli and fry for 1-2 minutes
5. Add the turmeric and ground coriander and cook for 20 seconds. Add the tomato puree and mix well
6. Add the yogurt, mix thoroughly with the other ingredients and heat through gently
7. Once the aubergine and tomatoes are cooked cut them into pieces and mix through the curry sauce. Cook for a further 5 minutes stirring occasionally

8. Serve with wedges of lime to squeeze over.

Cook's Tip: If you don't like aubergines, you can use fennel or Romanesco cauliflowers. Try using some fresh Thai basil as a garnish.

©2022 ALLIANCE FOR NATURAL HEALTH INTERNATIONAL

SAVOURY GRAM PANCAKES

Rainbow Rating

INGREDIENTS:

- 130 g gram (chickpea) flour
- 200 ml water
- 2 tbsp extra-virgin olive oil, plus more for cooking
- ½ tsp Himalayan or sea salt
- 1 tsp za'atar or ¼ tsp ground cumin (optional)

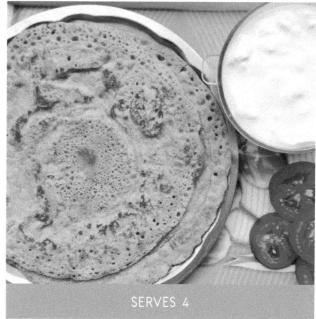

SERVES 4

METHOD:

1. Whisk the chickpea flour, water, olive oil, and salt together in a medium bowl until smooth
2. Leave to rest for 30 minutes to give the flour time to absorb the water
3. Heat a medium frying pan and add oil
4. Add a ladle of batter to the pan and swirl to coat the bottom of the pan
5. Cook until bottom is set and edges are starting to brown
6. Flip carefully to cook underside
7. Slide onto a plate and continue to cook more pancakes until all the mixture is used.

Cook's Tip: These are absolutely delicious and can be served with any of your favourite fillings. Experiment with dhal, pestos, houmous variations, crushed pea with pinenuts and halloumi strips, guacamole and peppers…. You get the idea!

Rainbow Rating

F4H

STIR-FRIED TEMPEH WITH BEAN SPROUTS AND COCONUT

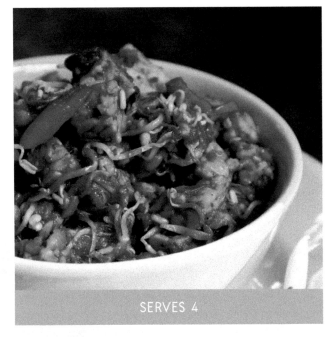

SERVES 4

V

VE

INGREDIENTS:

- 1 tbsp olive oil
- 1 tsp mustard seeds
- 1 tsp nigella seeds
- Thumb sized piece of fresh root ginger cut into small batons or grate for a less gingery hit
- 2 cloves garlic sliced
- 1 tsp ground turmeric
- Ground chilli to taste
- 2 tbsp desiccated coconut
- 250 g tempeh
- 400 g bean sprouts
- Sea salt or Himalayan pink salt & ground black pepper
- Chopped fresh coriander to garnish
- Tamari to serve

METHOD:

1. Add the oil to a non-stick pan/wok and heat gently
2. Add the mustard and nigella seeds and cook until they start to pop (around 1 minute)
3. Stir in the ginger and garlic and cook for 1 minute
4. Add the turmeric and chilli powder and mix well
5. Add the coconut and stir well
6. Add the tempeh and stir-fry on low to medium heat for at least 20 mins, add the bean sprouts for the last couple of minutes
7. Season to taste with tamari, salt and pepper
8. Sprinkle with the fresh chopped coriander and serve.

Cook's Tip: You may need to add a little water or tamari if you find your tempeh sticking whilst it's cooking.

©2022 ALLIANCE FOR NATURAL HEALTH INTERNATIONAL

KICKSTARTER RECIPES:

DINNER

CAN BE MADE VEGAN

Rainbow Rating

F4H

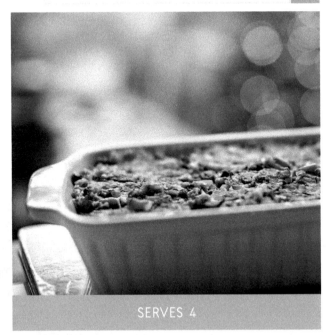

SERVES 4

ALMOND AND SESAME NUT ROAST WITH ONION GRAVY

INGREDIENTS:

*   2 tbsp extra virgin olive or coconut oil
*   1 large red or white onion finely chopped
*   ¼ cup risotto rice
*   1 ¼ cups vegan vegetable stock
*   1 large carrot grated
*   1 large leek trimmed and finely chopped
*   2 tsp sesame seeds, toasted
*   ¾ cup flaked almonds, toasted
*   ½ cup ground almonds
*   1 cup vegan / cheddar cheese, chopped very small or grated
*   2 tsp egg replacer mixed with 4 tbsp water or 2 eggs
*   1 tsp fresh rosemary finely chopped (or dried if fresh not available)

*   2 tsp fresh oregano finely chopped (or dried if fresh not available) - can substitute for 5 tsp dried Italian herbs if necessary
*   2 tsp fresh thyme finely chopped (or dried if fresh not available) (can substitute for 5 tsp dried Italian herbs if necessary)
*   1 tsp salt
*   ½ tsp ground black pepper

Onion Gravy

*   1 large onion
*   1 ¼ cups vegetable stock
*   ½ tbsp balsamic vinegar
*   1 tsp mustard powder or vegan mustard of your choice
*   2 tbsp olive oil
*   1 tablespoon cornflour to thicken
*   Salt and pepper to taste

©2022 ALLIANCE FOR NATURAL HEALTH INTERNATIONAL

METHOD:

1. Toast almonds in oven and sesame seeds in a dry fry pan, stirring until golden, and set aside
2. Heat oil in a large pan and fry the onion gently for 2-3 minutes
3. Add the risotto rice and cook slowly for 5-6 minutes stirring frequently
4. Add the stock to the onion, cornflower, mustard powder mix stirring all the time as you gently bring up the heat
5. Add the vegetable stock bring to a boil and then simmer for about 15 minutes or until the rice is tender
6. Add extra water as necessary. Remove from the heat and transfer to a large mixing bowl. Add the carrot, leek, sesame seeds, almonds (flaked and ground), vegan / cheddar cheese, egg replacer / eggs and herbs to the mixture
7. Mix well and season with salt and pepper
8. Transfer the mixture to a greased loaf tin, taking care to level the top
9. Bake in a preheated oven at 180°C/350°F for about 1 hour until set and firm. The loaf should be browned and crispy on the top but take care not to burn
10. Leave to cool in the loaf tin for 10 minutes before turning out onto a serving dish.

Onion Gravy

1. Make the gravy by sautéing the chopped onions in the olive oil until properly cooked and browned on the edges to caramelise
2. Sprinkle in the cornflour and stir until dissolved
3. Sprinkle on the mustard powder until dissolved
4. Add the balsamic vinegar to the stock a little at a time, stirring continuously
5. Bring to the boil stirring constantly until thickened and blended. Season to taste with salt and pepper
6. Cut the nutroast into slices and pour over the onion gravy
7. Garnish with some fresh, chopped herbs.

CAN BE MADE VEGAN

Rainbow Rating

F4H

ASIAN CAULIFLOWER RICE STIR FRY

SERVES 4

INGREDIENTS:

- 1 head of cauliflower
- 150 g green beans, sliced
- 6 spring onions, sliced
- 1 clove garlic, crushed
- 5 cm fresh ginger, peeled and grated
- Half a head of broccoli, sliced
- 2 pak choi, roughly chopped
- 1 small onion, chopped
- 2 carrots, finely sliced
- 1 yellow pepper
- 1 small pkt baby corn

- 2 eggs, lightly beaten (if tolerated), with salt and pepper
- 2 tbsp chopped fresh coriander
- 2 tbsp Thai basil
- A handful of beansprouts
- 2 tbsp coconut oil
- 1 tsp sesame oil
- 4 tbsp gluten-free Tamari
- 100 g cashew nuts (if tolerated)
- Salt and pepper to taste, but do taste before adding

METHOD:

1. Blitz the raw cauliflower florets in a food processor or Vitamix and put the 'rice' to one side
2. Preheat the oven to 220°C/450°F, when up to temperature, place the cashew nuts on a baking tray and bake for 7 mins or until lightly browned and crispy - take care not to burn! Set aside
3. Heat the coconut oil in a large frying pan or wok and add the onion, garlic, ginger, broccoli, pak choi stem (white part), carrots, yellow pepper and baby corn to the pan. Add the tamari and stir fry for approx. 5 minutes until just tender, but still crunchy. It's fine to add a bit of water if it's looking too dry. Once tender, but with some crunch, add the chopped herbs and combine
4. Add the cauliflower rice, pak choi leaves (green part) and bean sprouts. Mix well on a high heat until the rice is hot and well mixed through. Add more Tamari to taste as needed
5. If using eggs, make a well in the centre of the frying pan and pour in the beaten egg mixture. Allow a minute or two to cook and then mix through the stir fry
6. Just before serving add the cashew nuts and fresh coriander.

If you like your food spicy, then add as much chilli as you like during the cooking stage!

You can add whatever vegetables you like so don't be limited, experiment away.

 ©2022 ALLIANCE FOR NATURAL HEALTH INTERNATIONAL

BAKED EGGS

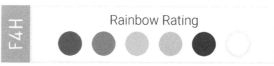

Rainbow Rating

INGREDIENTS:

- 8 eggs
- 1 large handful of fresh coriander, leaves and stalks roughly chopped

For the tomato sauce

- 1 tbsp olive oil
- 1 large onion, diced
- 2 garlic cloves, finely diced
- 1 orange bell pepper, diced
- 1 tbsp ground cumin
- 1 tsp smoked paprika
- Finely diced fresh red chilli, to taste
- 2 x 400 g tins of tomatoes
- 2 tbsp tomato puree
- 8 large handfuls of spinach, roughly chopped
- Sea salt and black pepper to taste

For the guacamole

- 2 large ripe avocados
- Juice 1 lime
- 2 spring onions, chopped
- 1 handful of fresh coriander leaves, chopped
- ½ fresh chilli, finely chopped (optional)
- Sea salt to taste

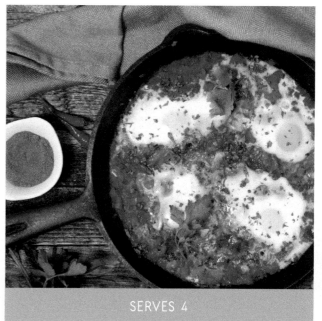

SERVES 4

METHOD:

Make the guacamole

1. Scoop out the avocado flesh from the shells and place in a bowl
2. Mash with a fork
3. Add the juice of the lime, spring onions, coriander leaves, salt and chilli if using
4. Mix well
5. Cover and leave in fridge
6. Preheat the oven to 180°C fan/ 350°F.

Make the tomato sauce

1. Heat oil in a large pan
2. Add the diced onion and pepper and cook for 5-6 minutes until they start to soften.
3. Add the garlic, cumin and paprika and cook for a further minute
4. Add the tinned tomatoes, tomato puree, spinach and chilli
5. Stir well
6. Simmer on a low heat for 5 minutes to allow the flavours to develop
7. Season with salt and pepper to taste
8. Put the tomato sauce in a large ovenproof dish (or divide between two smaller ones)
9. Make 8 wells then crack an egg into each well
10. Bake in the oven until the whites of the egg are set, but the yolks are soft
11. Scatter the chopped coriander over the top.

Serve with the guacamole.

©2022 ALLIANCE FOR NATURAL HEALTH INTERNATIONAL

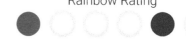

BAKED TEMPEH

F4H

Rainbow Rating

● ○ ○ ○ ● ○

V

VE

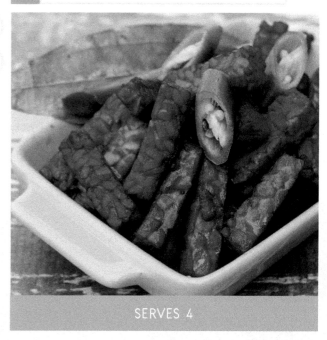

SERVES 4

INGREDIENTS:

- 450 g tempeh
- 1 cup cloudy apple juice
- ¼ cup shoyu soya sauce or tamari
- 2 tbsp rice wine vinegar
- 60 ml virgin olive oil

- 2 tbsp mirin
- Ground chilli to your taste
- 2 garlic cloves, crushed
- Himalayan pink salt and ground black pepper to taste

METHOD:

1. Cut the tempeh into 2 cm / 1 inch cubes
2. Prepare the marinade. Put the apple juice, shoyu/tamari, vinegar, oil, mirin, chilli powder, garlic, salt and pepper into a bowl and whisk thoroughly
3. Add the tempeh to the marinade and leave to marinate for at least 30 minutes
4. Preheat the oven to 180°C/350°F
5. Put the tempeh cubes in a shallow baking dish in a single layer
6. Pour the marinade over the tempeh
7. Bake for 30-40 minutes (until most of the marinade has been absorbed) and the tempeh is golden brown.

Cook's Tip: Shoyu sauce is usually gluten-free, but if you're concerned, then switch to tamari instead. Note the use of tempeh instead of tofu, as it's fermented and much easier on the gut. The omnivores can substitute the tempeh for chicken mini fillets or sliced beef.

VEGAN

Rainbow Rating

F4H

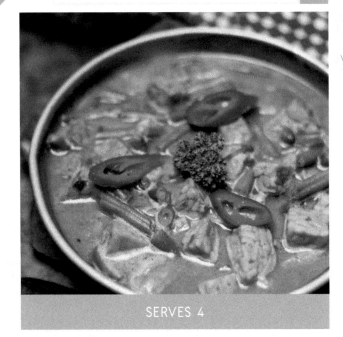

SERVES 4

V

VE

BRAISED TEMPEH
WITH CURRIED COCONUT SAUCE

INGREDIENTS:

- 450 g tempeh
- 300 ml water
- 60 ml apple juice or mirin
- 60 ml tamari
- 4 cm piece of fresh ginger, unpeeled, cut into 6 pieces
- 2 tsp curry powder
- 1 tsp paprika

Curried Coconut Sauce

- 1 tbsp coconut oil or extra-virgin olive oil
- 1 medium onion, finely diced
- 2 cloves garlic, crushed

- 400 g can coconut milk (full fat)
- 2 tsp curry powder
- ¼ tsp garam masala
- ½-1 tsp chilli powder (to taste)
- Himalayan pink salt and ground black pepper to taste
- 1 tsp fresh lemon juice

120 g dried unsweetened desiccated/shredded coconut for garnish

METHOD:

1. Cut the tempeh into pieces
2. Put them in a pan with the water, apple juice (or mirin if using), tamari, ginger pieces, curry powder and paprika. Cover and bring to a boil. Lower the heat and simmer for 15 minutes. Remove the tempeh and set it aside

3. Make the sauce by warming the oil in a medium frying pan over a medium to low heat. Add the onions and garlic and fry until golden (approx. 5 mins), then add the spices and lemon juice and cook for around 20 secs. Add the coconut milk, stir well to incorporate the spices, heat gently then season to taste

4. Serve the tempeh, topped with the sauce and garnished with desiccated/shredded coconut.

©2022 ALLIANCE FOR NATURAL HEALTH INTERNATIONAL

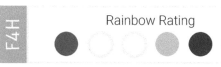

COCONUT CAULIFLOWER 'RICE' WITH SAMBAL AND OKRA

Rainbow Rating

F4H

INGREDIENTS:

- 600 g okra trimmed
- Large handful roughly chopped coriander for serving
- 2 limes, halved
- 150 g roasted cashew nuts

Sambal

- 5 fresh red chillies deseeded
- 5 dried red chillies deseeded
- 100 g baby shallots peeled or 1 small red onion
- 1 clove garlic, peeled
- ½ tsp pink Himalayan salt
- 130 ml olive oil
- 2 tbsp water
- ½ tbsp tamarind paste or 1 tbsp thick tamarind water (mix tamarind pulp with water and then strain)
- 1 tbsp coconut sugar (or you can use caster sugar)

Rice

- 325 g cauliflower 'rice'
- ½ tsp salt
- 175 ml tinned coconut milk (full fat)
- 350 ml water
- 6 kaffir lime leaves (optional)
- 6 thin slices of fresh root ginger

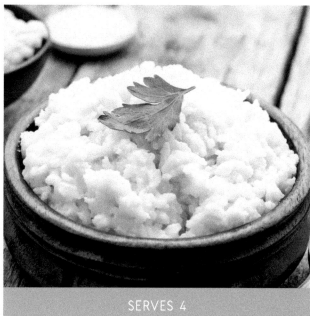

SERVES 4

Cook's Tip: If you don't like too much chilli use less of the sambal and add a bit of water to stretch it. For omnivores, this recipe goes particularly well with any Asian-style chicken dish.

METHOD:

1. Heat the oven to 180°C fan/ 200°C/400°F. Put the cashews on a baking tray and make sure they lie in one layer. Roast until just browning, but check frequently so as not to burn them. Stir or shake the pan a few times to even the colour. Place to one side once roasted

2. Make the sambal: place the chillies, shallots (or onion), garlic and salt in a food processor with 2 tbsp of the oil and the water and blitz for approx. 1 minute or until you get a fine paste

3. Heat a frying pan or wok to a high heat. Once hot add the remaining oil and heat before adding the chilli paste and stir

4. Reduce to a low heat to avoid burning the paste and cook on a low simmer, stirring frequently, for 5-10 minutes or until you get a lovely dark-red oily paste

5. Remove the paste from the heat and stir in the tamarind paste or water and sugar. Put to one side

6. Blitz the cauliflower into rice in a food processor and transfer to a medium saucepan with the salt, coconut milk, water, lime leaves and ginger. Stir and bring to the boil. Reduce to a simmer and cook for 12 minutes. Cover with a lid, then remove from the heat and leave to stand for 10 minutes. Stir the cauliflower rice with a fork before serving

7. While the rice is cooking, add the okra to boiling water and boil for 2-3 minutes. Drain then rinse under cold running water to stop the cooking process

8. Add the okra to the pan with the sambal paste, stir well and warm through

9. On a large plate or platter, serve the 'rice' topped with the okra and sprinkled with the roasted cashews and chopped fresh coriander. Lastly, squeeze the lime juice across the dish and enjoy.

©2022 ALLIANCE FOR NATURAL HEALTH INTERNATIONAL

HERBY MINCE

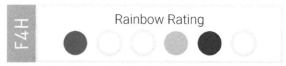

Rainbow Rating

INGREDIENTS:

- 400 g minced/ground beef, chicken or pork
- 2 red onions
- 3 sticks celery
- 2 large carrots
- 200 g frozen peas
- 6 blocks frozen spinach
- 2 tbsp each of chopped sage,

oregano and rosemary
- 3 large cloves garlic
- 3 tbsp olive oil
- 2 cubes of beef stock or gels
- 1 tsp red wine or apple cider vinegar
- Salt and pepper to taste

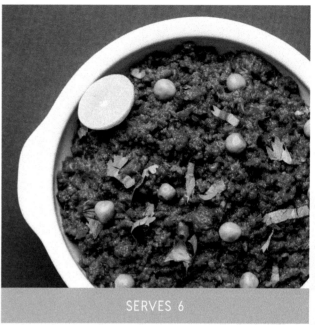

SERVES 6

METHOD:

1. Peel and chop the onions, celery and carrots, place in a large saucepan or deep-sided frying pan with a lid and add the garlic, crushed
2. Fry the onions and veg in the olive oil until the onions are transparent
3. Add the minced/ground meat, break it up and keep moving it around the pan to make sure it mixes with the vegetables and browns evenly (about 3-5 mins)

4. Add the fresh herbs, crumbled stock cubes or stock gels and mix well
5. Pour over 150 ml boiling water, tsp of vinegar and add the frozen spinach
6. Put a lid on and fast simmer for 15 mins, stirring from time to time to make sure it doesn't stick
7. Add salt and pepper to taste and the frozen peas. Put the lid back on and simmer for a further 5 mins until the peas are defrosted and hot.

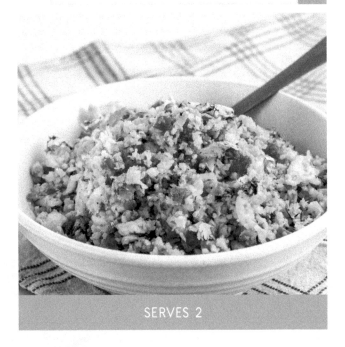

Rainbow Rating

F4H

SERVES 2

KEDGEREE WITH A DIFFERENCE

INGREDIENTS:

- 4 white fish fillets (about 350 g)
- 1 large head of cauliflower
- 2 white onions
- 1 large bag of curly parsley, chopped
- A handful of chopped coriander
- 2 bay leaves

- 1 rounded tsp curry powder (optional)
- 4 eggs - hard boiled and cooled
- 150 g frozen peas
- Salt and coarse black pepper to taste
- 50 g butter or 2 tbsp olive oil

METHOD:

1. Place the fish in a saucepan with the bay leaves, cover with water and bring to the boil. Then simmer for around 8 mins till poached. Set the water aside in a jug and cover the fish
2. Blitz the cauliflower head in a food processor to make fine grains, or chop very small
3. Peel and chop the onions, fry gently in half the butter or oil until transparent
4. Add the curry powder and fry for about a minute
5. Add the cauliflower 'rice' and saute until cooked, about 5-6 mins - if it's too dry at this stage add a bit of the fish stock, but not too much
6. Add the frozen peas after 3 mins
7. Once the cauliflower is cooked, flake the fish and add to the 'rice' along with the sliced or cubed hard-boiled eggs
8. Stir through the chopped parsley and coriander and salt and pepper to taste
9. Drop knobs of the remaining butter on the top or drizzle with the oil and stir to mix through, put a lid on the pan and make sure it's properly hot before serving.

©2022 ALLIANCE FOR NATURAL HEALTH INTERNATIONAL

RICH LENTIL STEW

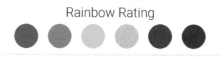

Rainbow Rating

CAN BE MADE VEGAN

INGREDIENTS:

- 3 tbsp coconut or olive oil
- 1 large onion, finely chopped
- 2 sticks celery, diced
- 1 leek, cut in half lengthways and diced
- 2 carrots, diced
- 1 large courgette diced
- ¼ small head of red cabbage, finely sliced
- 5 garlic cloves, finely chopped
- 1 tsp ground cumin
- 1 tsp ground coriander
- 1 tsp turmeric powder
- ¼ – ½ tsp hot chilli powder
- 300 g puy lentils (or 2 tins cooked lentils)
- 2 L chicken, beef or vegetable stock
- 1 400 g tin chopped tomatoes
- 2 tbsp tomato puree
- 2 tbsp fresh coriander as a garnish
- Salt and pepper to taste
- 250-300 g spinach or kale

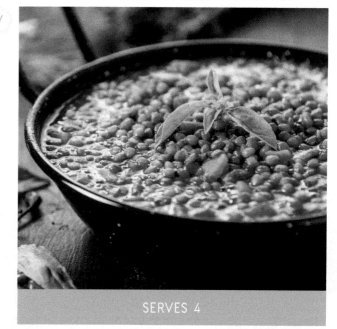

SERVES 4

METHOD:

1. In a large, heavy bottomed pan heat the oil and sauté the onion, celery, leek, carrot, courgette, cabbage and garlic for 10 minutes to soften
2. Add the spices and cook for a couple of minutes then add the lentils, stock, tomatoes and tomato puree
3. Bring to the boil, lower the heat and simmer for 30-40 minutes until the lentils are soft, stirring occasionally
4. Add a little more water or stock if it's too thick. Season, then add the spinach (or kale), cook until it's wilted.

Cook's Tip: If you have a pressure cooker you can save time and make sure your lentils are lectin-free.

CAN BE MADE VEGAN

Rainbow Rating

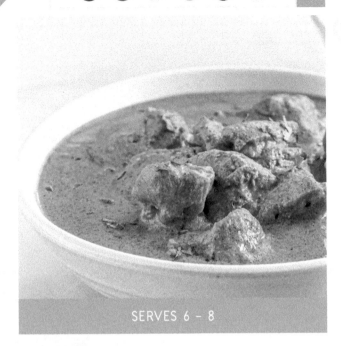

SERVES 6 – 8

v

SOUTH EAST ASIAN CHICKEN / VEGETABLE CURRY

INGREDIENTS:

- 1 kg diced (organic) chicken thighs or cubed butternut squash
- 2 onions, diced
- 6 kaffir lime leaves
- 1 cinnamon stick
- 4 star anise
- 1 tin coconut milk
- 500 ml chicken / veg stock
- 3 tbsp coconut oil
- 1 tsp palm sugar
- 2 tbsp gluten-free Tamari
- 2 tbsp fish sauce (omit if making vegetarian option)
- A large handful of fresh coriander, chopped, for garnish
- ½ lime
- 1 small can coconut cream

For the curry paste:

- 3 cloves garlic, crushed
- 2 lemon grass stalks (crush between 2 boards to break the outer surface)
- 1 red chilli, deseeded, chopped (more if you like it hot!)
- 1 lime, juiced
- 2 cm chunk of peeled ginger, grated
- 1 tbsp turmeric
- ½ tbsp ground coriander
- ¼ tbsp garam masala

©2022 ALLIANCE FOR NATURAL HEALTH INTERNATIONAL

METHOD:

1. Fry the onions, chilli and garlic gently in the coconut oil until slightly softened, then add the ingredients for the curry paste and continue frying till the onions are translucent
2. Add the chicken and continue frying for 2-3 mins to seal. If you're using butternut cubes, add them once all the other ingredients are in as they take less time to cook
3. Add the liquid ingredients - stock, coconut milk, Tamari and fish sauce (omit the fish sauce if making a vegetarian version)
4. Add the lime leaves, the star anise and cinnamon stick
5. Stir in 1 tsp palm sugar and combine well. Add the butternut cubes at this point if using
6. Chicken - bring to the boil then simmer on a very low heat for 2 hours or more. The chicken should be melt in the mouth soft
7. Butternut - bring to the boil and then simmer on a very low heat until soft
8. Just before serving stir in the lime juice, the can of coconut cream (minus the water) and the chopped fresh coriander.

NB: Add only as much stock as you need to cover the chicken, but don't flood the dish as you don't want to be left with a watery dish at the end. This curry is best when made the day before leaving it to stand overnight to let the flavours develop.

Serve with coconut rice and a crunchy salad laced with fresh coriander.

Can freeze and reheat, but you'll need to add more coconut cream to bring it all together before serving.

CAN BE MADE VEGAN

Rainbow Rating

F4H

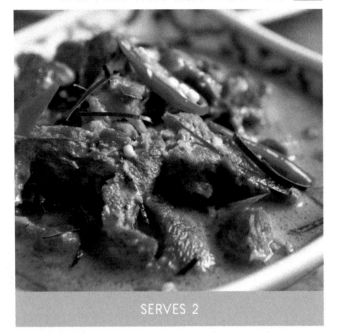

SERVES 2

THAI CURRY WITH BEEF

INGREDIENTS:

- 2 tbsp coconut oil
- 6 spring onions, finely sliced (keep 2 for garnish)
- 4 medium-sized mushrooms, thinly sliced (optional)
- 4 broccoli florets, thinly sliced
- 2.5 cm fresh ginger, peeled and roughly chopped
- 1 clove of garlic, crushed
- 1 small stick of lemongrass, cut into chunks
- 2 tsp of ground cumin
- 1 lime leaf (fresh is best)
- 1 lime, juiced

- 350 g beef, sliced into batons (or tempeh cubes)
- 400 g tin coconut milk
- 100 ml beef (or vegetable) stock
- 100 g baby spinach
- ½ red chilli, de-seeded and roughly chopped (more if you like it hot!)
- Bunch of fresh coriander, chopped (keep some for garnish)
- Himalayan pink salt

METHOD:

1. Ahead of cooking: Prepare the curry paste by adding the ginger, garlic, chilli, lemongrass, lime leaf, cumin, half the lime juice, 1 tbsp coconut oil, coriander and 2 tbsp of coconut milk to a small food processor or use a pestle and mortar. Add ¼ tsp of salt. Blend to form a chunky paste. Coat the beef batons in the curry paste and leave to marinate for at least 30 mins at room temperature
2. Heat the remaining 1 tbsp of coconut oil in a saucepan over a medium to high heat
3. Remove the sliced beef from the marinade with a slotted spoon and sear on all sides for 2-3 mins, turn the heat down, add the rest of the marinade and gently heat until fragrant
4. Add the remaining coconut milk and the stock, a little at a time to make sure the sauce doesn't become too thin
5. Add the sliced mushrooms, if using, and the sliced broccoli, bring to a gentle boil and reduce immediately to an open simmer (no lid) for 8-10 minutes, checking you don't overcook the veg
6. Taste and add more salt if needed
7. Once the broccoli is cooked through but still green, remove the pan from the heat and stir through the spinach until just wilted and the rest of the lime juice
8. Scatter with the remaining spring onions, extra coriander and some slices of fresh red chilli. Serve with the rice of your choice.

Cook's Tip: Serve with cauliflower or broccoli rice if you're going keto/low carb. Vegans and vegetarians can switch the beef for tempeh cubes but follow the same recipe. If using a pestle & mortar, make sure you chop everything as finely as you can before grinding as it will take far less elbow grease to make the paste!

©2022 ALLIANCE FOR NATURAL HEALTH INTERNATIONAL

FOOD4HEALTH MASALA

Rainbow Rating

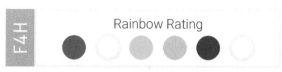

INGREDIENTS:

- 1 medium onion, finely chopped
- 2 cloves garlic, crushed
- 2 tbsp ghee or coconut oil
- 400 g boneless fish (e.g. salmon, cod), cut into bite-sized pieces
- 1 tbsp ground turmeric
- 2 tsp ground coriander
- 2 tsp ground cumin
- ¼ tsp asafoetida or 2 cloves garlic, crushed
- 2 cm (1 inch) piece of fresh ginger grated
- 1 red chilli, finely chopped
- Himalayan salt to taste
- 200 g baby spinach leaves

- 4 fresh tomatoes skinned, deseeded and chopped
- 350 g broccoli florets
- 300 g green beans chopped in 2.5 cm lengths
- 115 ml creamed coconut
- Juice of 1/4 lime (or lemon)
- 100 g skin on almonds, toasted and roughly chopped
- 100 g walnuts toasted and roughly chopped
- 2 tbs fresh coriander stems, finely chopped
- 2 tbsp fresh coriander leaves, chopped

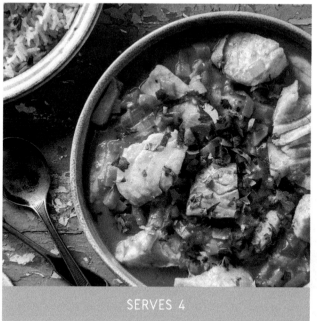

SERVES 4

METHOD:

1. Gently melt the ghee or coconut oil in a frying pan over a low heat and stir in the ground spices. Add the asafoetida (if using), onion, garlic, ginger, coriander stems and chilli along with a pinch of salt
2. Heat and stir for 2 minutes over a medium heat
3. Add fish pieces, turn them over in masala until covered and simmer gently for 3 minutes
4. Slowly add the spinach and stir until wilted. Add the tomatoes, broccoli and beans, put a lid on the pan and simmer for 3-4 minutes until the beans and broccoli are still bright in colour, but just tender
5. Stir through the creamed coconut, heat for a couple of minutes and season to taste
6. Transfer to a serving dish, drizzle with lime (or lemon) juice and sprinkle with the chopped nuts and coriander.

Cook's Tip: Serve with Basmati rice, which has lower glycaemic index, or cauliflower/broccoli rice if your intent is to go more keto.

*For additional health benefits for the mind and memory, add ½ tsp shankhpushpi (Convolvulus pluricaulis) powder and ½ tsp Brahmi (Bacopa monnieri) powder with other ground spices.

VEGAN

Rainbow Rating

F4H

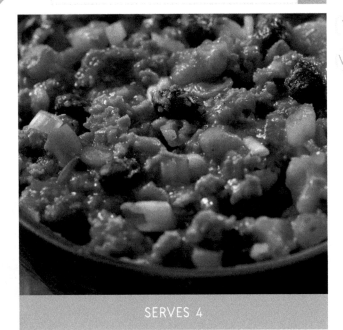

SERVES 4

V

VE

WALNUT CHILLI

INGREDIENTS:

- 2 tbsp extra virgin olive oil
- 5 stalks celery finely diced
- 2 cloves garlic crushed
- 1 medium onion, diced
- 1½ tsp ground cinnamon
- 2 tsp chilli powder (or to taste)
- 4 tsp ground cumin
- 1½ tsp smoked paprika
- 2 green bell peppers finely diced
- 2 courgettes diced
- 225 g mushrooms finely diced (optional)
- 1½ tbsp tomato puree
- 400 ml can chopped tomatoes
- 600 ml water
- 200 ml coconut milk (full fat)
- 350 g tempeh cut into pieces
- 200 g walnuts chopped
- 1 tbsp unsweetened cacao powder or cocoa powder
- Himalayan pink salt and ground black pepper

To serve:

- Chopped fresh coriander
- 1 ripe avocado, sliced
- 2 tbsp radishes, finely sliced

METHOD:

1. Heat the oil in a large pot over medium heat. Add the celery and onion and cook for 4-5 minutes. Add the garlic, cinnamon, chilli powder, cumin and paprika and stir until fragrant, about another 2 minutes
2. Add the peppers, courgette and mushrooms, if using, and cook for 5 minutes
3. Add the tomato puree, tomatoes, water, coconut milk, walnuts and cacao/cocoa powder
4. Reduce the heat to medium-low and simmer for about 20-25 minutes until thick and the vegetables are soft
5. Add the tempeh and warm through
6. Season with salt and pepper, to taste.
7. Serve topped with avocado, radishes, and coriander.

©2022 ALLIANCE FOR NATURAL HEALTH INTERNATIONAL

CHILDREN'S SNACKS

Rainbow Rating

● ● ● ● ●

SAVOURY BAKED FLAPJACKS

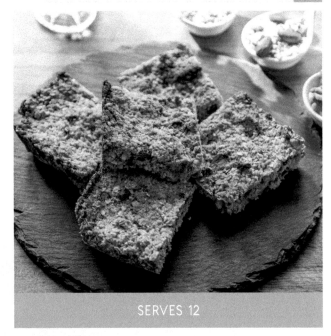

SERVES 12

INGREDIENTS:

Makes a good side for soup!

- 150g porridge oats
- 150g mature cheddar / hard cheese, grated or 3 tbsp Marigold Swiss Vegetable Bouillon Powder (if going dairy free)
- 1 large carrot
- 1 large courgette
- 1 large red onion
- 2 tbsp each of pumpkin and sunflower seeds
- 150g chopped nuts e.g. almonds and walnuts
- 1 tbsp each of fresh chopped sage, oregano, thyme
- and rosemary
- 2 large eggs (or 3 if you're making the dairy-free version), beaten
- 50g butter or 3 tbsp extra virgin olive oil or deodorised coconut oil (if going dairy free)
- Sea salt and pepper to taste

METHOD:

1. Preheat the oven to 180°C/350°F
2. Grease a square or rectangular baking tray with deep sides with butter or oil
3. Finely chop the carrot, courgette and onion or blitz in a food processor
4. Finely chop or blitz the nuts making sure you stop before they become powder. You still want a bit of crunch!
5. Put the oats, seeds, chopped veggies, nuts and herbs into a large mixing bowl
6. Add the grated cheese (or herb bouillon powder if going dairy-free) and mix thoroughly
7. Taste a bit of the mixture before adding salt and pepper to taste - or any other herbs or spices. If you're using the vegetable bouillon powder instead of the cheese, you'll need to add less salt
8. Add the beaten eggs, butter (melt first) or oils and mix well
9. Spoon the mixture into the baking tray and press down a little for an even, firm consistency
10. Grate some more cheese over the top or sprinkle parmesan and paprika and put into the oven to bake for around 35-40 mins. Ovens vary greatly, so please keep checking from 30 mins to make sure you don't burn the top
11. It's important to cut the flapjacks in the tin whilst hot, but leave in the tin to fully cool.

©2022 ALLIANCE FOR NATURAL HEALTH INTERNATIONAL

SAVOURY BHAJI BITES

VEGAN

F4H

Rainbow Rating

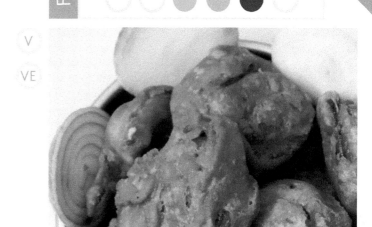

SERVES 6

V

VE

INGREDIENTS:

- 115 g gram flour (chickpea flour)
- 1 tsp baking powder
- ½ tsp ground cumin
- 1 tsp ground coriander
- 1 tsp ground turmeric
- 150 ml cold water
- 1 medium onion (finely sliced) or 50 g defrosted frozen peas or 1 small courgette grated
- Coconut oil for frying

METHOD:

1. Mix the first ingredients in a bowl. Then add the water and mix well to form a batter (double cream consistency)
2. Add your veg and mix well
3. Heat some oil in a frying pan over a medium heat. Cook spoonfuls of the mixture until golden then turn over and cook until golden on other side
4. Drain on kitchen paper
5. These keep well in the fridge or can be frozen (if frozen they benefit from a quick refresh in a warm frying pan once defrosted).

VEGAN

Rainbow Rating ● ●

F4H

V

VE

SWEET BHAJI BITES

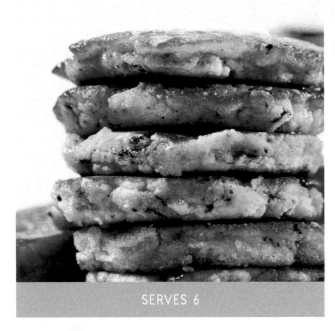

SERVES 6

INGREDIENTS:

- 115 g gram flour (chickpea flour)
- 1 tsp baking powder
- 1 tsp ground cinnamon
- 1 tsp vanilla paste
- 150 ml milk of choice (or water)
- 35 g sultanas
- Coconut oil for frying

METHOD:

1. Mix the first 3 ingredients in a bowl. Then add the liquid and mix well to form a batter (double cream consistency)
2. Add the sultanas and mix through well
3. Heat some oil in a frying pan over a medium heat
4. Cook spoonfuls of the mixture until golden then turn over and cook until golden on other side
5. Drain on kitchen paper
6. These keep well in the fridge or can be frozen (if frozen they benefit from a quick refresh in a warm frying pan once defrosted).

©2022 ALLIANCE FOR NATURAL HEALTH INTERNATIONAL

NO RECIPE REQUIRED!

Boiled eggs with spinach or rocket or baby tomatoes

Boil half a dozen eggs and keep in the fridge for when needed during the week

Oatcakes

Topped with hummus or nut butter

Houmous with veg crudités

Apple or pear sarnies

Two thick slices apple or pear with core removed, spread with nut butter, sandwich together

Celery sticks

Filled with nut butter of choice or hummus topped with raisins or cranberries

Handful of preferred berries topped with coconut cream

Handful of nuts with a piece of fruit

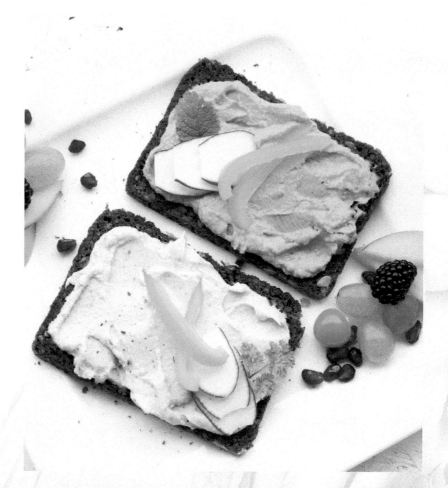

SIMPLE SIDES

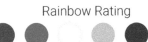

Rainbow Rating

● ● ○ ● ● ○

F4H

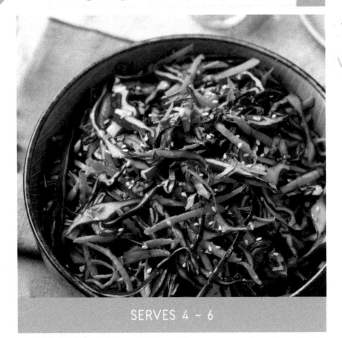

V

VE

SERVES 4 – 6

ANYTHING GOES SLAW

INGREDIENTS:

For the Slaw:

- ½ red, white or green cabbage finely shredded, blanched - or better still, all 3!
- 1 medium courgette grated
- 1 small raw beetroot grated
- ½ head of fennel finely sliced
- Medium carrot grated
- 1 apple grated (cored, leave skin on)
- 100 g chopped walnuts

For the dressing:

- 5 tbsp extra virgin olive oil
- 1 tbsp tahini
- A dash of maple syrup
- 3 tbsp lemon juice
- Salt & pepper to taste

The veg listed are our suggestion, you can use any combination of raw or lightly blanched veg, fruit and nuts you prefer

METHOD:

1. Place all the dressing ingredients in a bowl and whisk together
2. Mix the vegetables in another bowl season, add the dressing and mix together well.

©2022 ALLIANCE FOR NATURAL HEALTH INTERNATIONAL

VEGAN

BEAUTIFUL BEETROOT HOUMOUS

F4H

Rainbow Rating

INGREDIENTS:

- 1 can of chickpeas, drained and rinsed or 220 g cooked
- 100 g cooked and diced beetroot
- ½ tbsp lemon / lime juice
- 1 tsp (level) smoked / normal paprika
- 1 rounded tsp cumin
- 2 tbsp extra virgin olive oil
- ½ tbsp tahini
- 1 garlic clove, crushed or finely chopped
- A dash of Tabasco or Worcestershire sauce
- Pink salt and ground black pepper

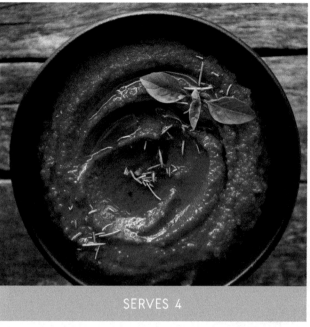

SERVES 4

METHOD:

1. Add ingredients to a blender and blend till smooth and creamy. You may need to add some additional water to get the consistency smooth and creamy
2. Mix this recipe up by using spinach and kale instead of beetroot or roasted peppers and carrots. You can also use harissa or chipotle instead of paprika. Experiment away!

VEGAN

Rainbow Rating

F4H

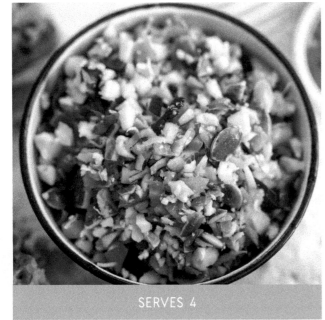

V

VE

SERVES 4

BROCCAULI TABBOULEH

INGREDIENTS:

- ½ head each cauliflower & broccoli, blanched
- 1 bunch of spring onions, finely chopped
- a handful of fresh mint leaves, finely chopped
- a handful of other fresh herbs as preferred (sorrel, basil, thyme, coriander, marjoram, oregano, lemon balm etc)
- 2 tbsp fresh pomegranate seeds

For the dressing:

- 1 tbsp pomegranate molasses
- 1 tbsp tahini
- 1 tsp maple syrup or runny honey
- 3 tbsp extra virgin olive oil
- 2 handfuls mixed pumpkin & sunflower seeds
- sea salt and black pepper

METHOD:

Use your favourite fresh herbs to bring this simple salad alive.

1. Break up the cauliflower & broccoli and blitz in a food processor into rice like pieces (you may need to do this in batches)
2. Chop the herbs and spring onions, add to the broccoli & cauliflower mixture along with the seeds and mix through well
3. Make the dressing by whisking the tahini, pomegranate molasses, olive oil, honey, salt and pepper together, taste to check
4. Pour the dressing over the salad, mix thoroughly and scatter with pomegranate seeds.

©2022 ALLIANCE FOR NATURAL HEALTH INTERNATIONAL

BROCCOLI SALAD

 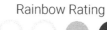 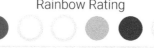

Rainbow Rating

INGREDIENTS:

- 450 g broccoli
- 100 g spring onions, sliced
- 100 g almonds, chopped
- 75 g light tahini
- Juice of 2 limes
- 2 tbsp sesame oil
- 2 cloves garlic crushed
- 1 green or red chilli finely diced (to taste)
- 3 tbsp tamari
- Himalayan pink salt and ground black pepper

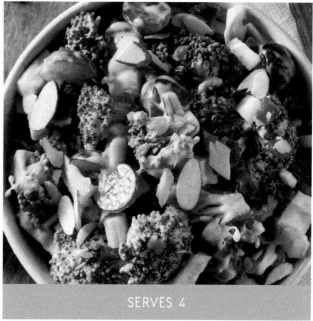

SERVES 4

METHOD:

1. Chop the broccoli into florets and steam for 5 minutes
2. Drain the broccoli and refresh under cold water
3. Mix the oil, tahini, lime juice, garlic, tamari and chilli together to make a dressing and season to taste
4. Put the steamed broccoli into a bowl and cover with the dressing, mixing well to coat the broccoli pieces
5. Sprinkle with the chopped almonds and spring onions.

Cook's Tip: add a combination of nuts and seeds to increase the levels of protein and healthy fats.

VEGAN

Rainbow Rating

F4H

V

VE

BUCKWHEAT AND CHIA SEED BREAD

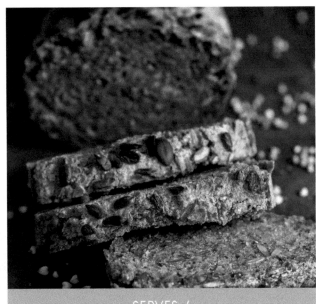

SERVES 4

INGREDIENTS:

- 300 g raw buckwheat - soaked for 2 hours till soft
- 60 g chia seeds
- 300 ml water (use half to soak the chia seeds for 30 mins and the other half for the blender mixture)
- ¼ cup olive oil
- ½ tsp baking powder
- ½ tsp salt

METHOD:

1. Pre-heat the oven to 160°C/320°F
2. Oil and line a loaf tin
3. Drain the buckwheat, rinse and put in a blender/food processor. Add the chia gel, the remaining water, olive oil, baking powder and salt. Blend until you have a smooth batter consistency
4. Pour into the loaf tin and bake for 1 hour and 15 mins until it's firm to the touch and bounces back
5. Cool in the tin for 30 mins on a rack before turning out.

Cook's Tip: You may need a little more water if your mixture is too solid. It's good to set some whole buckwheat aside to add back in so you have some crunch in your bread. Alternatively, you can add in some nuts and seeds to the batter before baking. Try some dried cranberries, sour cherries or apricot pieces for a little extra tang.

©2022 ALLIANCE FOR NATURAL HEALTH INTERNATIONAL

CAJUN SWEET CORN RELISH

VEGAN

F4H

Rainbow Rating

V

VE

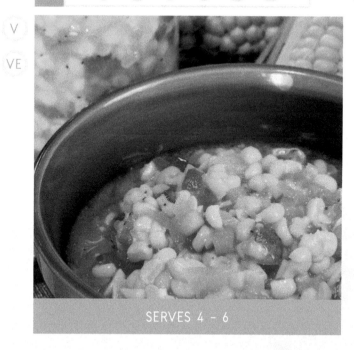

SERVES 4 – 6

INGREDIENTS:

- 400 g fresh corn kernels
- 1 tbsp extra-virgin olive oil
- 1 medium red onion, finely diced
- ½ green bell pepper, finely diced
- 2 tomatoes, diced
- 1 tsp Cajun spice mix
- Himalayan pink salt and ground black pepper

METHOD:

1. Put half the corn kernels into a blender with 50ml of water and purée until smooth
2. Warm the oil in a medium frying pan, add the onions and bell peppers and sauté over a medium-low heat for about 7 minutes
3. Add the tomatoes and cajun spice, then cook for a few minutes until they're soft
4. Stir in the corn purée and cook for another 5 minutes stirring constantly
5. Season with salt and pepper
6. Serve hot or cold.

VEGAN

Rainbow Rating

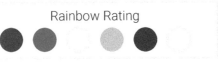

F4H

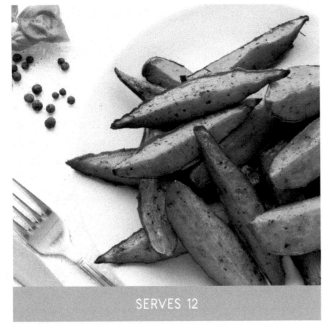

SERVES 12

CAJUN SWEET POTATO WEDGES

V

VE

INGREDIENTS:

- 500 g skin-on sweet potatoes, well-scrubbed and cut into wedges
- 1 tbsp ground black pepper
- 1 tbsp paprika/chipotle
- 1 tsp cayenne pepper

- A pinch of chilli powder (optional)
- 3 tbsp fresh chopped herbs or 1 tbsp dried mixed herbs
- Pink sea salt

METHOD:

1. Preheat the oven to 200°C/400°F
2. Lightly coat the wedges with olive oil
3. Mix the herbs, spices, salt and pepper in a bowl, add the wedges and coat them well with the mixture
4. Place on a baking tray in the oven for 20-30 mins until crisp and golden on the outside

5. They should still be soft and squishy on the inside. Use them as dipping sticks or on their own.

©2022 ALLIANCE FOR NATURAL HEALTH INTERNATIONAL

CAULI UPMA

VEGAN

F4H

Rainbow Rating

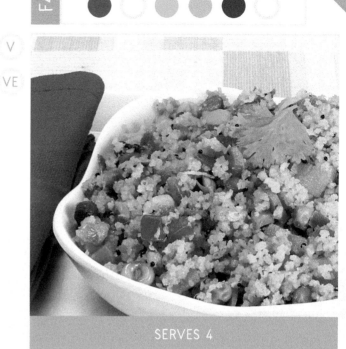

V

VE

SERVES 4

INGREDIENTS:

- 100 g cauliflower
- 100 g broccoli
- 3 tbsp ghee (if tolerated) or coconut oil
- 100 g cashew nuts
- 10 g grated fresh ginger
- 60 g hemp hearts
- 1 large red onion diced
- 400 ml water

- 6-8 curry leaves
- 2 tbsp cumin seeds
- 2 tbsp mustard seeds
- 1 green chilli finely chopped
- 1 tbsp ground turmeric
- Himalayan pink salt and ground black pepper
- Fresh coriander for garnish

METHOD:

1. Blitz the cauliflower and broccoli in a food processor until it resembles rice. You may need to do this in batches, but make sure you remove them before they become a paste!
2. Add the cumin and mustard seeds to a dry pan and gently heat, moving them around so they don't burn. As soon as you start to smell the spice aroma, add the ghee or oil and heat
3. Once the seeds start to sizzle add the onion, curry leaves, chilli, turmeric and ginger. Season with salt and pepper
4. Fry the onions and spices until the onions are translucent
5. Add the cauliflower and broccoli and stir well to coat in the spices. Add the water
6. Cover and simmer for approx. 10 minutes, stirring regularly until the cauliflower and broccoli is just tender
7. Stir in the hemp hearts and sprinkle with fresh chopped coriander before serving.

Cook's Tip: Can be made with just cauliflower or broccoli.

VEGAN

Rainbow Rating

CHIMICHURRI

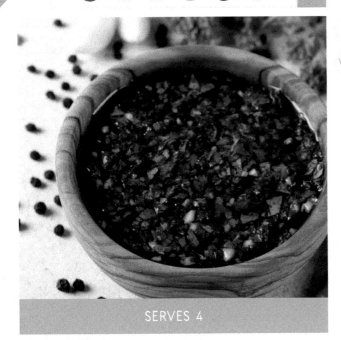

SERVES 4

V

VE

INGREDIENTS:

- ½ cup coarsely chopped flat-leaf parsley (ideally fresh, including stems)
- ¼ tablespoon oregano
- 3 tablespoons red/white wine or apple cider vinegar
- 4 large garlic cloves, minced (2 ½ tablespoons)
- 2 teaspoons finely chopped red (bell) pepper

- Salt and freshly ground black pepper
- ½ cup extra-virgin olive oil

A traditional South American sauce often used with grilled meat but that can be added to veg as well!

METHOD:

1. Finely chop the parsley and oregano. Add the vinegar, garlic and chopped red pepper
2. Season with salt and pepper. Transfer the sauce to a bowl and pour the olive oil over the mixture, mix well. Let it stand for at least 20 minutes. Can be made ahead and refrigerated overnight. Bring to room temperature before serving. Can also be used as a marinade.

Variations: This sauce is a great way to get more powerful herbs and spices into your diet. Mix it up with additions/ substitutions such as paprika, cumin, thyme, lemon, basil, coriander (cilantro), basil or sage. In its red version, tomato may also be added and for those of you who like a little more spice, add some chopped chilli peppers.

PESTO

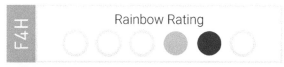

INGREDIENTS:

- 1 large bunch basil leaves
- 3 medium cloves of garlic
- 1 small handful raw pine nuts
- ¾ cup Parmesan, grated
- A few tablespoons of extra virgin olive oil

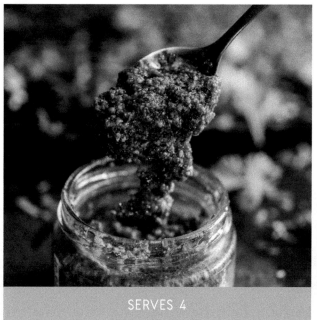

SERVES 4

METHOD:

1. If you have a food processor, throw in all the ingredients and blend
2. It's just as easy to make by hand. Mince or crush the garlic. Chop the basil. Chop the pine nuts. Mix the garlic, basil and pine nuts together with the Parmesan. Add the oil and mix well.

Variations: If you're dairy free omit the cheese or use a dairy-free alternative. Mix it up with basil, coriander (cilantro), rocket (arugula) or watercress and replace the pine nuts with walnuts or almonds. Really the variations are endless, so just experiment!

HEALTHY TREATS

CAN BE MADE VEGAN

Rainbow Rating

● ○ ○ ○   ● ● ●

F4H

ANYTIME PROTEIN BAR

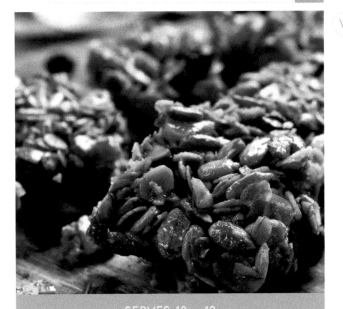

SERVES 10 – 12

INGREDIENTS:

- 90 g flaked almonds
- 90 g pecan nuts
- 60 g desiccated coconut
- 4 tbsp almond, cashew or peanut butter
- 4 tbsp extra virgin coconut oil
- 4 tbsp ground almonds
- 1.5 tsp vanilla extract
- 1 tsp honey or maple syrup
- 2 scoops protein powder (avoid whey)
- 1 large egg (optional)
- ½ tsp sea salt

- 125 g dried raspberries or blueberries
- Some extra desiccated coconut for the topping

METHOD:

1. Preheat the oven to 180°C/350°F and toast the nuts and desiccated coconut to a golden brown finish. You will need to mix the tray contents at least once whilst baking, which also helps you to ensure they don't burn!
2. Once toasted pour into a food processor and pulse till the mixture is coarsely ground. Turn the oven down to 160°C/320°F as soon as you take the mixture out and allow to cool to the new temperature

3. In a Bain Marie (glass bowl over hot water in a saucepan) heat the coconut oil and nut butter and stir together until smooth
4. Add the vanilla extract, honey and sea salt and mix thoroughly. Whilst still over the heat, fold in the nut mixture and protein powder, mix thoroughly
5. Add in the beaten egg and mix thoroughly
6. Fold in the raspberries/blueberries or dark chocolate chips, mix thoroughly

7. Use coconut oil to thoroughly grease a brownie tin. Press the mixture into the tin and even it out
8. Place in the oven at 160°C/320°F for around 10 mins, but keep checking so it doesn't burn
9. Remove from the oven, sprinkle liberally with desiccated coconut and put it under the grill until the top just begins to turn brown
10. Allow to cool for 15-20 mins before you cut into slices ready for storing in an airtight container. This should make about 10-12 slices.

©2022 ALLIANCE FOR NATURAL HEALTH INTERNATIONAL

VEGAN

AVOCADO, LIME & COCONUT CRUMBLE POTS

Rainbow Rating

INGREDIENTS:

- 2 large very ripe avocados
- Grated zest and juice of 2 limes
- 3 tbsp coconut oil melted
- 3 tsp maple syrup
- 20 g desiccated coconut
- 10 g sunflower seeds
- 10 g ground almonds

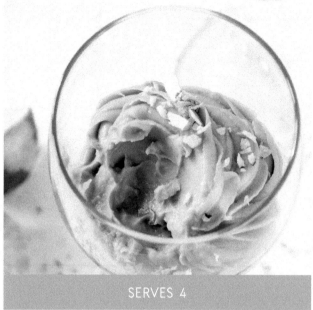

SERVES 4

METHOD:

1. Scoop out the flesh of the avocados and put in a processor. Add the lime juice, coconut oil, maple syrup and half the coconut and whizz until smooth
2. Divide the mixture between 4 ramekins and pop in the fridge for 2-4 hours to firm up
3. Mix the remaining coconut, sunflower seeds, ground almonds and lime zest then sprinkle over the top of each pot
4. Serve!

VEGAN

Rainbow Rating

⚪ ⚪ ⚪ ⚪ ⚫ ⚫

F4H

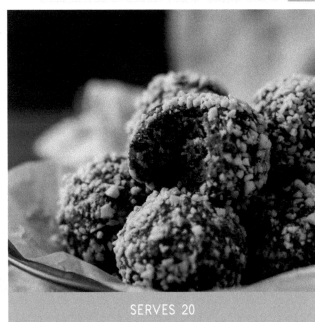

V

VE

SERVES 20

CHOCOLATE KETO BOMBS

INGREDIENTS:

- 220 g Coconut Oil
- 220 g Almond Butter
- 32 g Coconut Flour
- 15 g Cacao Powder
- 150 g Raw Cashews

METHOD:

1. In a non-stick medium saucepan over medium heat, heat coconut oil and almond butter stirring to mix evenly
2. Pour the oil mixture from the pan into a bowl and mix in coconut flour and cacao powder
3. Place bowl in the freezer for about 15 minutes until mixture cools and is solid
4. While the mixture is cooling, place the cashews in a food processor and pulse lightly for a chopped texture
5. When the coconut mixture is solidified, take ½ tablespoon of the mixture from the bowl, roll into a ball, and dip in the blended cashews
6. Place the Keto Bombs on a plate and repeat until you have used all of the mixture
7. Refrigerate all the Keto Bombs for at least 5 minutes before serving
8. Enjoy!

Cook's Tip: It's highly unlikely you will have any left, but if you do, make sure to store leftovers in the fridge, otherwise they will melt quickly.

©2022 ALLIANCE FOR NATURAL HEALTH INTERNATIONAL

DAIRY-FREE EGG CUSTARD

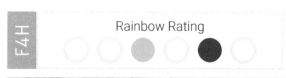

Rainbow Rating

INGREDIENTS:

- 4 egg yolks
- 1 litre dairy-free milk e.g. oat, or other plant-based milk of your choice
- 2 tbsp corn flour
- 2 tbsp xylitol
- 1 tbsp erythritol
- 1 vanilla pod or 1 tbsp vanilla essence

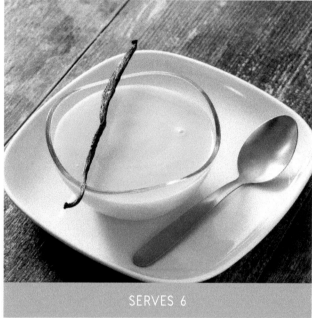

SERVES 6

METHOD:

1. Scrape the inside of the vanilla pod into the dairy-free milk, or add the vanilla essence and gently heat in a large saucepan. Bring to almost boiling point
2. In a bowl whisk the egg yolks with the cornflour, xylitol and erythritol till light, white and creamy
3. When the milk is almost boiling, remove from the heat and add to the bowl whisking all the time to mix thoroughly and prevent the cornflour from going into lumps
4. Return the custard to the saucepan and gently heat again stirring continuously to prevent lumps, but don't let it boil
5. The custard is ready once hot and fully thickened in ~5 mins.

VEGAN

Rainbow Rating

F4H

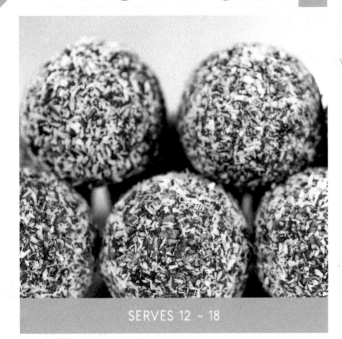

SERVES 12 – 18

V

VE

GOLDEN BLISS BALLS

INGREDIENTS:

- 270 g Apricots
- 150 g Cashews (or other nuts of choice)
- 2 tbsp Tahini
- Desiccated coconut for rolling
- 1 scoop vanilla protein powder of choice (optional)

METHOD:

1. Put the nuts into a food processor and blitz into fine pieces
2. Put the nuts into a bowl
3. Add the apricots to the processor and blend until smooth (you will need to keep stopping and scraping down the sides of the bowl)
4. Add the nuts and tahini to the processor with the apricots and blend until incorporated
5. Roll into approx 2cm (1 inch) balls
6. Roll in the desiccated coconut
7. Pop into the fridge to firm up.

©2022 ALLIANCE FOR NATURAL HEALTH INTERNATIONAL

NO CHEESE BERRY 'CHEESECAKE'

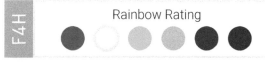

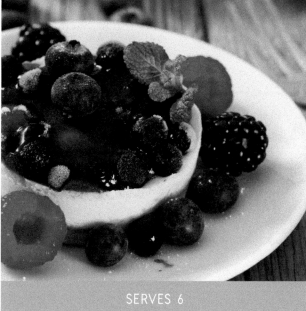

Rainbow Rating

F4H

SERVES 6

INGREDIENTS:

- 400 g cashew nuts, soaked overnight ideally or min 4 hours
- Olive oil for greasing the tin
- 2 tbsp desiccated coconut
- 3 lemons, juiced
- 2 limes, juiced
- ½ cup maple syrup
- 2 tsp vanilla extract
- 180 ml coconut oil, melted

For the base:

1. Either use a pre-baked gluten-free pastry base, or
2. Use the following, which will increase the sugar content:

- 150 g Medjool pitted dates
- 150 g ground almonds
- 1 scoop protein powder (avoid whey!) - optional
- 100 g hazelnuts or pecans
- 1 – 2 tbsp melted coconut oil (add slowly until desired consistency)
- Small pinch of salt

For the polyphenol-rich berry coulis top:

- 250 g frozen mixed berries
- ½ sliced cooking apple
- ½ lemon, juiced
- 1 tbsp palm sugar
- 2 tbsp water

METHOD:

If using dates: Place in warm water and soak for 20 mins, or until soft. Drain, add to a food processor and blitz. When blended to a paste, add the ground almonds, hazelnuts or pecans, protein powder (if using) and oil. Blend until combined in a crumble consistency. Press into the base of the prepared flan dish or pie pan.

1. Grease a flan dish or pie tin with the olive oil and sprinkle liberally with the desiccated coconut to help it not to stick
2. In a food processor or Vitamix add the drained and rinsed cashews, the coconut oil, the lemon and lime juice, maple syrup and vanilla extract
3. Blend until combined in to a creamy, thick consistency
4. Taste and add more maple syrup to your taste
5. Pour the mixture over the base and place in the fridge for 3-4 hours if you have time, or the freezer for 45 mins.

For the polyphenol-rich berry coulis top:

1. Place all the ingredients in a small saucepan and bring to the boil
2. Turn down and simmer until the consistency becomes like jam and all the berries have broken down. You may need to squash some with a spoon!
3. Turn off the heat and allow to cool
4. Once cool to the touch, pour over the set cheesecake and return to the fridge or freezer until the top is set
5. Sprinkle with more desiccated coconut and serve with coconut yoghurt.

©2022 ALLIANCE FOR NATURAL HEALTH INTERNATIONAL

PARADISE SQUARES

Rainbow Rating
○ ○ ○ ○ ● ●

CAN BE MADE VEGAN

INGREDIENTS:

- 200 g bar of creamed coconut
- 6 tbsp softened coconut oil
- 2 tbsp raw honey or maple syrup
- 150 g desiccated coconut

- 1½ tsp vanilla extract or paste
- Pinch of sea salt
- 100 g (70%+ cocoa solids) dark chocolate (any flavour of your choice)

V

VE

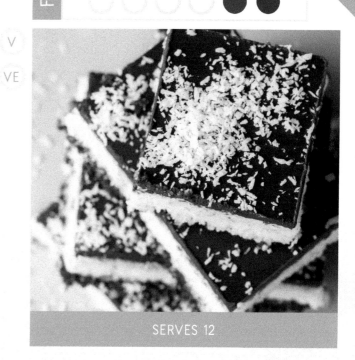

SERVES 12

METHOD:

1. Line a 20cm (7" or 8") square tin with baking parchment. Place the unopened packet of creamed coconut in a bowl of warm water to soften
2. Once the creamed coconut is soft all the way through pour it into a bowl with the softened coconut oil, honey, vanilla and salt and mix well
3. Mix in the desiccated coconut evenly to create a stiff consistency

4. Pour the mixture into the lined tin. Press mixture down with the back of a spoon so it's level and leave to set in fridge
5. Melt the chocolate in a glass bowl over a pan of warm water
6. Spread the melted chocolate over the top of the coconut mixture and pop back into the fridge to set
7. Once set leave to come up to room temperature and cut into squares
8. Keeps well in the fridge or freezer.

EPILOGUE

In the pause before you eat...

By adapting our lifestyles to the demands of our lives, while finding ways to function at our optimum, we also make a huge contribution to the sustainability of the health systems around us. Sustainability in healthcare – a concept that the Alliance for Natural Health, the organisation we represent, has pioneered, has a large element of personal responsibility. We need to consider sustainability in health, as much as we do with our environment, because healthcare systems are buckling under the stress of preventable disease.

It's also about understanding the potential impact of our behaviours and choices on our health and on society more widely. With an understanding of the causes of disease — not just a knowledge of how to treat symptoms — we put ourselves in a strong position to create health and prevent the descent into full-blown diseases. However, if disease and ill health is your current reality, take heart.

Our bodies have a miraculous ability to heal and regenerate once we give them what they need. Using food and lifestyle changes to 'inform' different gene expression is the most powerful medicine on the planet. And it's within the grasp of each of us.

As we move into a world in which the biggest burdens on health systems globally are ones that are entirely preventable, we need to take responsibility for our own health. We can't simply make it someone else's problem, like our doctor's, and then demand a 'pill for my ill'. That model may have worked in the early days of antibiotics in combatting the infectious diseases of the day. But it doesn't work for the 21st century epidemic of chronic, degenerative and autoimmune diseases that most people battle with during the latter one-third or so of their lives.

Let's not give up on science, on nature, on each other, or on the future. The current challenges we face are even more of a reminder that change lies in our hands. It's an exciting time to be alive and between us, we can make a difference.

Eating well isn't some unobtainable goal. Our Food4Health Guidelines can help you unlock a brighter, more vital, optimally healthy life!

We look forward to partnering you on your Health Creation journey.

Rob Melein

Melissa

There is a wealth of additional information that's constantly updating and expanding at www.anhinternational.org. Please sign up for our free weekly newsletter and join our burgeoning community of Health Creators!

Fats

Lichtenstein AH, Ausman LM, Jalbert SM, et al. Effects of different forms of dietary hydrogenated fats on serum lipoprotein cholesterol Levels. **NEJM.** 1999; 340:1933-1940.

Ascherio A, Katan MB, Zock PL, et al. Trans fatty acids and coronary heart disease. **NEJM.** 1999; 340: 1994-1998.

Berglund L. HDL-subpopulation pattern in response to reductions in dietary total and saturated fat intakes in healthy subject. **Am J Clin Nutr.** 1999; 70: 992-1000.

Broadhurst CL, Cunnane SC, Crawford MA. Rift Valley lake fish and shellfish provided brain-specific nutrition for early homo. **Brit J Nutr.** 1998; 79: 3-21.

Broadhurst CL. Balanced intakes of natural triglycerides for optimum nutrition: an evolutionary and phytochemical perspective. **Med Hypoth.** 1997; 49: 247-261.

Brouwer DA, Hettema Y, van Doormaal JJ, et al. Alpha-linolenic Acid does not augment long-chain polyunsaturated fatty acid omega-3 status. **Prostaglandins Leukot Essent Fatty Acids.** 1998; 59(5): 329-334.

De Lorgeril M, Renaud S, Mamelle N, et al. Mediterranean alphalinolenic acid-rich diet in secondary prevention of coronary heart disease. **The Lancet.** 1994; 343: 1454-1459.

De Lorgeril M, Salen P, Martin JL, et al. Effect of a Mediterranean type of diet on the Rate of cardiovascular Complications in Patients with coronary artery disease. **JACC.** 1996; 28(5): 1103-1108.

Dreon DM, Fernstrom HA, Williams PT, et al. A very-low-fat diet is not associated with improved lipoprotein profiles in men with a predominance of large, ion-density lipoproteins. **Am J of Clin Nutr.** 1999; 69: 411-418.

Harcombe Z, Baker JS, DiNicolantonio JJ, et al. Evidence from randomised controlled trials does not support current dietary fat guidelines: a systematic review and meta-analysis. **Open Heart.** 2016; 3(2): e000409.

Pan DA, Hulbert AJ, Storlien LH. Dietary fats, membrane phospholipids and obesity. **J Nutr.** 1994; 124: 1555-1565.

Ramsden CE, Faurot KR, Carrera-Bastos P, et al. Dietary fat quality and coronary heart disease prevention: a unified theory based on evolutionary, historical, global, and modern perspectives. **Curr Treat Options Cardiovasc Med.** 2009; 11(4): 289-301.

Ravnskov U. The Questionable role of saturated and polyunsaturated fatty acids in cardiovascular disease. **J Clin Epidemiol.** 1998; 51(6): 443-460.

Williams PT. Low-fat diets, lipoprotein subclasses and heart disease risk. **Am J Clin Nutr.** 1999; 70: 949-950.

Yam D, Eliraz A, Berry EM. Diet and disease - The Israeli Paradox: possible dangers of a high Omega-6 poly unsaturated fatty acid diet. Isr. **J Med Sci.** 1996; 32: 1134-1143.

Yehuda S, Rabinovitz S, Carasso RL, et al. Fatty Acids and Brain Peptides. **Peptides.** 1998; 19(2): 407-419.

Protein

Appel LJ, Sacks FM, Carey VJ, et al. Effects of protein, monounsaturated fat, and carbohydrate intake on blood pressure and serum lipids: results of the OmniHeart randomized trial. **JAMA.** 2005; 16;294(19):2455-64.

Gannon MC, Nuttall FQ, Saeed A, et al. An increase in dietary protein improves the blood glucose response in persons with type 2 diabetes. **Am J Clin Nutr.** 2003; 78(4):734-41.

Hoffman JR, Falvo MJ. Protein – Which is best? **J Sports Sci Med.** 2004; 3(3): 118–130.

Levey AS, Adler S, Caggiula AW, et al. Effects of dietary protein restriction on the progression of advanced renal disease in the modification of diet in renal disease study. **Am J Kidney Dis.** 1996; 27(5): 652-63.

Lonnie M, Hooker E, Brunstrom JM, et al. Protein for life: Review of optimal protein intake, sustainable dietary sources and the effect on appetite in ageing adults. **Nutrients.** 2018; 10(3): 360.

Lieb CW. The effects on human beings of a twelve month exclusive meat diet. **JAMA.** 1929; 93 (1): 20-22.

Joint FAO/WHO/UNU Expert Consultation on Protein and Amino Acid Requirements in Human Nutrition. Protein and amino acid requirements in human nutrition. 2002; **WHO Technical Report Series** 935.

Phillips SM, Van Loon LJC. Dietary protein for athletes: from requirements to optimum adaptation. **J Sports Sci.** 2011; 29 Suppl 1:S29-38.

Van der Kuil WA, Engberink MF, Brink EJ, et al. Dietary protein and blood pressure: a systematic review. **PLoS One.** 2010; 5(8): e12102.

Ketogenic

Carroll J, Koenigsberger D. The ketogenic diet: a practical guide for caregivers. **J Am Diet Assoc.** 1998; 98(3): 316-21.

Cassidy CM. **Nutrition and health in agriculturalists and hunter-gatherers: a case study of two prehistoric populations. In: Nutritional Anthropology: Contemporary Approaches to Diet & Culture.** Jerome NW, Kandel RF, Pelto GH (Eds). 1980. Pleasantville, NY: Redgrave Publishing Co.

©2022 ALLIANCE FOR NATURAL HEALTH INTERNATIONAL

Cohen MN. The significance of long-term changes in human diet and food economy. Food and Evolution. **Toward a Theory of Human Food Habits.** 1987. pp 261-283. University Press.

Cordain L, Eaton SB, Miller JB, et al. The paradoxical nature of hunter-gatherer diets: meat-based, yet non- atherogenic. **Eur J Clin Nutr.** 56 Suppl 1 2002; S42-52. Review.

Fleming J, Sharman MJ, Avery NG, et al. Endurance capacity and high-intensity exercise performance responses to a high fat diet. Int **J Sport Nutr Exerc Metab.** 2003; 13(4): 466-78.

Golay A, Eigenheer C, Morel Y, et al. Weight-loss with low or high carbohydrate diet? **Int J Obes.** 1996; 20: 1067-1072.

Grundy S. The Optimal ratio of fat-to carbohydrate in the diet. **Ann Rev Nutr.** 1999; 19: 325-341.

JS Volek, MJ Sharman, AL Gómez, DA, et al. Comparison of energy-restricted very low-carbohydrate and low-fat diets on weight loss and body composition in overweight men and women. **Nutr Metab.** (Lond). 2004; 1(1): 13.

Leite JO, DeOgburn R, Ratliff J, et al. Low-carbohydrate diets reduce lipid accumulation and arterial inflammation in guinea pigs fed a high- cholesterol diet. **Atherosclerosis.** 2010; 209(2): 442-8.

Leite JO, DeOgburn R, Ratliff JC, et al. Low-carbohydrate diet disrupts the association between insulin resistance and weight gain. **Metabolism.** 2009; 58(8): 1116-22.

Nebeling LC, Lerner E. Implementing a ketogenic diet based on medium-chain triglyceride in pediatric patients with Cancer. **J Am Diet Assoc.** 1995; 95: 693-697.

Paoli A, Rubini A, Volek JS, et al. Beyond weight loss: a review of the therapeutic uses of very-low-carbohydrate (ketogenic) diets. **Eur J Clin Nutr.** 2013; 67(8): 789-96.

Prasad AN, Stafstrom CA. Dietary Therapy of epilepsy in the nineties; renewed experience with the Ketogenic Diet. **Nutr Res.** 1998; 18(2): 403-416.

Rasmussen OW, Thomsen C, Hansen KW, et al. Effects on blood pressure, glucose and lipid levels of a high-monounsaturated fat diet compared with a high-carbohydrate diet in NIDDM subjects. **Diab Care.** 1993; 16: 1565-1571.

Feinman RD, Pogozelski WK, Astrup A, et al. Dietary carbohydrate restriction as the first approach in diabetes management: critical review and evidence base. **Nutrition.** 2015; 31(1): 1-13.

Sharman MJ, Kraemer WJ, Love DM, et al. A ketogenic diet favorably affects serum biomarkers for cardiovascular disease in normal-weight men. **J Nutr.** 2002; 132(7): 1879-85.

Sharman MJ, Volek JS. Weight loss leads to reductions in inflammatory biomarkers after a very-low-carbohydrate diet and a low-fat diet in overweight men. **Clin Sci (Lond).** 2004; 107(4): 365-9.

Sheard N. The Diabetic Diet: Evidence for a new approach. **Nutr Rev.** 1995; 53(I): 16-18.

Volek JS, Gómez AL, Kraemer WJ. Fasting lipoprotein and postprandial triacylglycerol responses to a low- carbohydrate diet supplemented with n-3 fatty acids. **J Am Coll Nutr.** 2000; 19(3): 383-91.

Noakes T, Volek JS, Phinney SD. Low- carbohydrate diets for athletes: what evidence? **Br J Sports Med.** 2014l ;48(14): 1077-8.

Volek JS, Noakes T, Phinney SD. Rethinking fat as a fuel for endurance exercise. **Eur J Sport Sci.** 2015; 15(1): 13-20.

Volek JS, Vanheest JL, Forsythe CE. Diet and exercise for weight loss: a review of current issues. **Sports Med**. 2005; 35(1): 1-9. Review.

Westman EC, Mavropoulos J, Yancy WS, et al. A review of low-carbohydrate ketogenic diets. **Curr Atheroscler Rep.** 2003; 5(6): 476-83. Review.

Westman EC, Yancy WS, Haub MD, et al. Insulin resistance from a low carbohydrate, high fat diet perspective. **Metab Syndr Relat Disord.** 2005; 3(1): 14-8.

Wood RJ, Fernandez ML, Sharman MJ, et al. Effects of a carbohydrate-restricted diet with and without supplemental soluble fiber on plasma low-density lipoprotein cholesterol and other clinical markers of cardiovascular risk. **Metabolism.** 2007; 56(1): 58-67.

Gluten

Catassi C, Bai JC, Bonaz B, et al. Non-Celiac Gluten sensitivity: the new frontier of gluten related disorders. **Nutrients.** 2013 Sep 26; 5(10): 3839-53. Review.

Catassi C, Kryszak D, Bhatti B, et al. Natural history of celiac disease autoimmunity in a USA cohort followed since 1974. **Ann Med.** 2010; 42(7): 530-8.

Cordain L. Cereal grains: humanity's double- edged sword. **World Rev Nutr Diet.** 1999; 84: 19-73. Review.

de Punder K, Pruimboom L. The dietary intake of wheat and other cereal grains and their role in inflammation. **Nutrients.** 2013; 5(3): 771-87.

Fasano A, Sapone A, Zevallos V, et al. Nonceliac gluten sensitivity. **Gastroenterology.** 2015; 148(6): 1195-204. Review.

Fasano A. Intestinal permeability and its regulation by zonulin: diagnostic and therapeutic implications. **Clin Gastroenterol Hepatol.** 2012; 10(10): 1096-1100.

Fasano A. Leaky gut and autoimmune diseases. **Clin Rev Allergy Immunol.** 2012 Feb; 42(1): 71-8.

Fasano A. Zonulin and its regulation of intestinal barrier function: the biological door to inflammation, autoimmunity, and cancer. **Physiol Rev.** 2011; 91(1): 151-75.

©2022 ALLIANCE FOR NATURAL HEALTH INTERNATIONAL

Fasano A. Zonulin, regulation of tight junctions, and autoimmune diseases. **Ann NY Acad Sci.** 2012; 1258: 25-33.

Hollon J, Puppa EL, Greenwald B, et al. Effect of gliadin on permeability of intestinal biopsy explants from celiac disease patients and patients with non-celiac gluten sensitivity. **Nutrients.** 2015; 7(3): 1565-76.

Jackson JR, Eaton WW, Cascella NG, et al. Neurologic and psychiatric manifestations of celiac disease and gluten sensitivity. **Psychiatr Q.** 2012; 83(1): 91-102. Review.

Pruimboom L, Fox T, Muskiet FA. Lactase persistence and augmented salivary alpha-amylase gene copy numbers might have been selected by the combined toxic effects of gluten and (food born) pathogens. **Med Hypotheses.** 2014; 82(3): 326-34.

Sapone A, Lammers KM, Casolaro V, et al. Divergence of gut permeability and mucosal immune gene expression in two gluten-associated conditions: celiac disease and gluten sensitivity. **BMC Med.** 2011; 9: 23

Schnedl WJ, Lackner S, Enko D, et al. Non-celiac gluten sensitivity: people without celiac disease avoiding gluten-is it due to histamine intolerance? **Inflamm Res.** 2018; 67(4): 279-284.

Dairy

Guggenmos J, Ogg S, Andersson M, et al. Antibody cross-reactivity between myelin oligodendrocyte glycoprotein and the milk protein butyrophilin in multiple sclerosis. **J Immunol.** 2004; 172(1):661-8.

Holden C, Mace R. Phylogenetic analysis of the evolution of lactose digestion in adults. **Hum Biol.** 1997; 69(5):605-28.

Lanou AJ. Should dairy be recommended as part of a healthy vegetarian diet? **Am J Clin Nutr.** 2009; 89(5): 1638S-1642S.

Laugesen M, Elliott R. Ischaemic heart disease, Type 1 diabetes, and cow milk A1 beta- casein. **N Z Med J.** 2003; 24; 116(1168): U295.

Mäkinen OE, Wanhalinna V, Zannini E, Ar. Foods for Special Dietary Needs: Non-dairy Plant-based Milk Substitutes and Fermented Dairy- type Products. **Crit Rev Food Sci Nutr.** 2016; 56(3):339-49.

Melnik BC, John SM, Schmitz G. Milk is not just food but most likely a genetic transfection system activating mTORC1 signaling for postnatal growth. **Nutr J.** 2013; 12:103.

Monetini L, Manfrini S, Stefanini L, et al. Antibodies to bovine beta-casein in diabetes and other autoimmune diseases. **Horm Metab Res.** 2002; 34(8):455-9.

Oldstone MBA. Molecular mimicry and immune-mediated diseases. **FASEB J.** 1998; 12(13): 1255-1265.

Otaegui D, Bernard CCA, Lopez-de- Munain A, et al. Increased transcriptional activity of milk-related genes following the active phase of experimental autoimmune encephalomyelitis and multiple sclerosis. **J Immunol.** 2007; 179(6):4074-82.

Sverrisdóttir OO, Timpson A, Toombs J, et al. Direct estimates of natural selection in Iberia indicate calcium absorption was not the only driver of lactase persistence in Europe. **Mol Biol Evol.** 2014; 31(4): 975-983.

Tishkoff SA, Reed FA, Ranciaro A, et al. Convergent adaptation of human lactase persistence in Africa and Europe. **Nat Genet.** 2007; 39(1):31-40.

Voskuil DW, Vrieling A, van't Veer LJ, et al. The insulin-like growth factor system in cancer prevention: potential of dietary intervention strategies. **Cancer Epidemiol Biomarkers Prev.** 2005; 14(1):195-203.

Zoghbi S, Trompette A, Claustre J, et al. β-Casomorphin-7 regulates the secretion and expression of gastrointestinal mucins through a μ-opioid pathway. **Mucos Biol.** 2006; 290(6): G1105-G1113.

Carb/insulin

Colagiuri S, Brand-Miller JC. The Metabolic Syndrome: from inherited survival trait to a health care problem. **Exp Clin Endocrinol Diab.** 1997; 105 suppl 2: 54-60.

Jenkins DJ, Wolever TM, Collier GR, et al. Metabolic effects of a low glycemic index diet. **Am J Clin Nutr.** 1987; 46: 968-975.

Eaton SB, Cordain L, Sparling PB. Evolution, body composition, insulin receptor competition, and insulin resistance. **Prev Med.** 2009; 49(4): 283-5. **Erratum in: Prev Med.** 2011; 52(1): 95.

Haffner SM. Epidemiology of type 2 diabetes: risk factors. **Diab Care.** 1998; 21 suppl 3: c3-6.

Hallberg SJ, McKenzie AL, Williams PT, et al. Effectiveness and safety of a novel care model for the management of type 2 diabetes at 1 Year: an open-label, non-randomized, controlled study. **Diabetes Ther.** 2018; 9(2): 583-612.

Holt S. Glycemic index, satiety and the cholecystokinin response. **Am J Clin Nutr.** 1994; 3(S): 787S.

Holt SH, Miller JC, Petocz P. An insulin index of foods: the insulin demand generated by 100 kJ portions of common foods. **Am J Clin Nutr.** 1997; 66: 1264-1276.

Kroemer G, López-Otín C, Madeo F, et al. Carbotoxicity — noxious effects of carbohydrates. **Cell.** 2018; 175(3): 605-614.

Ludwig DS, Majzoub JA, Al-Zahrani A, et al. High glycemic index foods, overeating and obesity. **Pediatrics.** 1999; 103(3): E26-E31.

Reaven G. Pathophysiology of insulin resistance in human disease. **Physiol Rev.** 1995; 3: 473-486.

Rossetti L. Glucose Toxicity. **Diab Care.** 1990; 13: 610-630.

Salmerón J, Manson JE, Stampfer MJ, et al. Dietary fiber, glycemic load, and risk of non-insulin-dependent diabetes mellitus in women. **JAMA.** 1997; 277: 472-477.

Trevisan R, Vedovato M, Tiengo A. The epidemiology of diabetes mellitus. **Nephrology, Dialysis Transplantation.** 1998; 13 suppl 8: 2-5.

©2022 ALLIANCE FOR NATURAL HEALTH INTERNATIONAL

Volek JS, Feinman RD. Carbohydrate restriction improves the features of Metabolic Syndrome. Metabolic Syndrome may be defined by the response to carbohydrate restriction. **Nutr Metab. (Lond).** 2005; 2: 31.

Caloric restriction

Blagosklonny MV. Once again on rapamycin-induced insulin resistance and longevity: despite of or owing to. **Aging.** 2012; 4(5): 350-358.

Fontana L, Klein S, O Holloszy J. Effects of long-term calorie restriction and endurance exercise on glucose tolerance, insulin actioFn, and adipokine production. **Age (Dordr).** 2010; 32(1): 97-100.

Stein K, Soare A, Meyer TE, et al. Caloric restriction may reverse age- related autonomic decline in humans. **Aging Cell.** 2012; 11(4): 644-650.

Gensous N, Franceschi C, Santoro A, et al. The impact of caloric restriction on the epigenetic signatures of aging. **Int J Mol Sci.** 2019; 20(8). pii: E2022.

Leclerk E, Trevizol AP, Grigolon RB et al. The effect of caloric restriction on working memory in health non-obese adults. **CNS Spectr.** 2020; 25(1): 2-8.

Paoli A, Tinsley G, Bianco A, et al. The influence of meal frequency and timing on health in humans: the role of fasting. **Nutrients.** 2019; 11(4). pii: E719.

Lectins

Barre A, Damme EJMV, Simplicien M, et al. Are dietary lectins relevant Allergens in plant food allergy? **Foods.** 2020; 9(12):1724.

Cordain L, Toohey L, Smith MJ, et al. Modulation of immune function by dietary lectins in rheumatoid arthritis. **Br J Nutr.** 2000; 83(3): 207-17. Review.

Gemede HF, Ratta N. Antinutritional factors in plant foods: potential health benefits and adverse effects. **Int J Nutr Food Sci.** 2014; 3(4): 284-289.

Gundry SR. **The Plant Paradox: The Hidden Dangers in "Healthy" Foods that Cause Disease and Weight Gain.** 2017. Harper Collins.

Lagarda-Diaz I, Guzman-Partida AM, Vazquez-Moreno L. Legume lectins: proteins with diverse applications. **Int J Mol Sci.** 2017; 18(6): 1242.

Lis H, Sharon N. Lectins. **Encyclopaedia of Immunology** (Second Edition). 1998. Academic Press. pp 1535-1541.

Lucius K. Dietary Lectins: gastrointestinal and immune effects. **Altern Complement Ther.** 2020; 26(4).

Peumans WJ, Van Damme EJM. Lectins as plant defense proteins. **Plant Physiol.** 1995; 109: 347-352.

Pellegrina CD, Perbellini O, Scupoli MT, et al. Effects of wheat germ agglutinin on human gastrointestinal epithelium: insights from and experimental model of immune/epithelial cell interaction. **Tox Appl Pharmacol.** 2009; 237: 146-153.

Samtiya M, Aluko RE, Dhewa T. Plant food anti-nutritional factors and their reduction strategies: an overview. **Food Prod Process and Nutr.** 2020; 2: 6.

Thakur A, Sharm V, Thakur A. An overview of anti-nutritional factors in food. **Int J Chem Stud.** 2019; 7(1): 2472-2479.

Vojdani A, Afar D, Vojdani E. Reaction of lectin-specific antibody with human tissue: possible contributions to autoimmunity. **J Immunol Res.** 2020: 1438957.

Yoo S-W, Motari MG, Susuki K, et al. Sialylation regulates brain structure and function. **FASEB J.** 2015; 29(7): 3040-53.

Phytonutrients/fibre

Axelsson AS, Tubbs E, Mecham B et al. Sulforaphane reduces hepatic glucose production and improves glucose control in patients with type 2 diabetes. **Sci Transl Med.** 14 2017; 9(394): eaah4477.

Dufour V, Stahl M, Baysse C. The antibacterial properties of isothiocyanates. **Microbiology.** 2015; 161(2).

Fiedor J, Burda K. Potential role of carotenoids as antioxidants in human health and disease. **Nutrients.** 2014; 6(2): 466-488.

Ganesan K, Jayachandran M, Xu B. A critical review on hepatoprotective effects of bioactive food components. **Crit Rev Food Sci Nutr.** 2018; 58(7): 1165-1229.

Higdon JV, Delage B, Williams DE, et al. Cruciferous vegetables and human cancer risk: epidemiologic evidence and mechanistic basis. **Pharmacol Res.** 2007; 55(3):224-236.

Huang M, Lu JJ, Huang MQ, et al. Terpenoids: natural products for cancer therapy. **Expert Opin Investig Drugs.** 2012; 21(12): 1801-18.

Jones JL, Fernandez ML, McIntosh MS, et al. A Mediterranean-style low-glycemic- load diet improves variables of metabolic syndrome in women, and addition of a phytochemical- rich medical food enhances benefits on lipoprotein metabolism. **J Clin Lipidol.** 2011; 5(3): 188-96.

Knekt P, Reunanen A, Järvinen R, et al. Antioxidant vitamin intake and coronary mortality in a longitudinal population study. **Am J Epidemiology.** 1994; 139: 1180-1189.

Navarro SL, Li F, Lampe JW. Mechanisms of action of isothiocyanates in cancer chemoprevention: an update. **Food Funct.** 2011; 2(10):579-87.

Ornish D. Can lifestyle changes reverse coronary heart disease? **The Lancet.** 1990; 336: 129-133.

Panche AN, Diwan AD, Chandra SR. Flavonoids: an overview. **J Nutr Sci.** 2016; 5:e47.

Russo GL, Spagnuolo C, Russo M, et al. Mechanisms of aging and potential role of selected polyphenols in extending healthspan. **Biochem Pharmacol.** 2020; 173: 113719.

Santino A, Scarano A, De Santis S, et al. Gut microbiota modulation and anti-inflammatory properties of dietary polyphenols in IBD: new and consolidated perspectives. **Curr Pharma Des.** 2017; 23(16).

©2022 ALLIANCE FOR NATURAL HEALTH INTERNATIONAL

Spiller GA, Jenkins DA, Bosello O, et al. Nuts and plasma lipids: an almond-based diet lowers LDL-C while preserving HDL-C. **J Am Coll Nutr.** 1998; 17(3): 285-290.

Vahid H, Rakhshandeh H, Ghorbani A. Antidiabetic properties of Capparis spinosa L. and its components. **Biomed Pharmacother.** 2017; 92: 293-302.

Verlangieri AJ, Kapeghian JC, el-Dean S, et al. Fruit and vegetable consumption and cardiovascular mortality. **Med Hypoth.** 1985; 16: 7-15.

Walk AM, Edwards CG, Baumgartner NW, et al. The role of retinal carotenoids and age on neuroelectric indices of attentional control among early to middle-aged adults. **Front Aging Neurosci.** 2017; 9:183.

Xiao ZP, Peng ZY, Peng MJ, et al. Flavonoids health benefits and their molecular mechanism. **Mini Rev Med Chem.** 2011; 11(2):169-77.

Dietary diversity & quality

Alkerwi A, Sauvageot N, Malan L, et al. Association between nutritional awareness and diet quality: evidence from the observation of cardiovascular risk factors in Luxembourg (ORISCAV-LUX) study. **Nutrients.** 2015; 7(4): 2823–2838.

Arimond M, Ruel MT. Dietary diversity is associated with child nutritional status: evidence from 11 demographic and health surveys. **J Nutr.** 2004; 134(10): 2579-85.

Bes-Rastrollo M, Basterra-Gortari F, Sánchez-Villegas A, et al. A prospective study of eating away-from-home meals and weight gain in a Mediterranean population: The SUN (Seguimiento Universidad de Navarra) cohort. **Publ Health Nutr.** 2010; 13(9): 1356-1363.

Edwards CA, Havlik J, Cong W, et al. Polyphenols and health: Interactions between fibre, plant polyphenols and the gut microbiota. **Nutr Bull.** 2017; 42(4): 356-360.

Elmadfa, I. Diet diversification and health promotion. **Forum Nutr.** 2005; 57: 147-156.

Jacobs DR, Gross MD, Tapsell LC, et al. Food synergy: an operational concept for understanding nutrition. **Am J Clin Nutr.** 2009; 89(5): 1543S-1548S.

Johns T, Eyzaguirre PB. Linking biodiversity, diet and health in policy and practice. **Proc Nutr Soc.** 2006; 65(2): 182-9.

Makki K, Deehan EC, Walter J, et al. The impact of dietary fibre on gut microbiota in host health and disease. **Cell Host Microbe.** 2018; 23(6): 705-715.

Kim S, Haines PS, Siega-Riz AM, et al. The Diet Quality Index-International (DQI-I) provides an effective tool for cross-national comparison of diet quality as illustrated by China and the United States. **J Nutr.** 2003; 133(11):3476-84.

Machado-Rodrigues AM, Gama A, Mourão I, et al. Eating away from home: a risk factor for overweight in children. **Eur J Clin Nutr.** 2018; 72: 1724–1727.

Moursi MM, Arimond M, Dewey KG, et al. Dietary diversity is a good predictor of the micronutrient density of the diet of 6- to 23-month-old children in Madagascar. **J Nutr.** 2008;138(12): 2448-53.

Brand-Miller JC, Mann NJ, Cordain L. Paleolithic nutrition: what did our ancestors eat? **Genes to Galaxies.** 2009 [online].

Kew Royal Botanical Gardens, 2017 State of the World's Plants. [online].

General

Bazzano LA, Hu T, Reynolds K, et al. Effects of low-carbohydrate and low-fat diets: a randomized trial. **Ann Intern Med.** 2014; 161(5): 309-18.

Cordain L, Boyd Eaton S, Sebastian A, et al. Origins and evolution of the Western diet: health implications for the 21st century. **Am J Clin Nutr.** 2005; 81(2): 341-54. Review.

Dehghan M, Mente A, Zhang X, et al. Associations of fats and carbohydrates with cardiovascular disease and mortality in 18 countries from five continents (PURE): a prospective cohort study. **The Lancet.** 2017; 390 (10107):2050-2062.

Diamond J. **The Third Chimpanzee: The Evolution and Future of The Human Animal.** 1992. pp 180-191. Harper Collins.

Eaton SB, Cordain L. Evolutionary aspects of diet: old genes, new fuels. Nutritional changes since agriculture. **World Rev Nutr Diet.** 1997; 81: 26-37. Review.

Eaton SB, Konner M. Paleolithic nutrition, a consideration of its nature and current implications. **N Engl J Med.** 1985; 312: 283-289.

Eaton SB, Eaton III Sb, Konner MJ. Paleolithic nutrition revisited: a twelve-year retrospective on its nature and implications. **Euro J Clin Nutr.** 1997; 51: 207-216.

Eaton SB, Konner M, Shostak M. Stone agers in the fast lane: chronic degenerative diseases in evolutionary perspective. **Am J Med.** 1988; 84: 739-749.

Enig M. Diet, serum Cholesterol and Coronary Heart Disease. In Mann GV (Ed) **Coronary Heart Disease.** 1993. Paul & Co Pub Consortium, USA.

Gkogkolou P, Böhm M. Advanced glycation end products. Key players in skin aging? **Dermatoendocrinol.** 2012; 4(3): 259–270.

Hallberg SJ, Gershuni VM, Hazbun TL, et al. Reversing type 2 diabetes: a narrative review of the evidence. **Nutrients.** 2019. 11(766).

Kanders BS, Blackburn GL: Reducing primary risk factors by therapeutic weight loss. In: **Treatment of the Seriously Obese Patient.** Wadden TA, Van Itallie TB (Eds). New York, Guilford, 1992 , pp. 213-230.

Milton K. Primate diet and gut morphology: Implications for hominid evolution. In Harris M. Ross EB: **Food and Evolution Philadelphia.** 1987. Temple University Press.

Mischoulon D, Fava M. Role of S-adenosyl-L-methionine in the treatment of depression: a review of the evidence. **Am J Clin Nutr.** 2002; 76(5): 1158S-61S.

©2022 ALLIANCE FOR NATURAL HEALTH INTERNATIONAL

O'Keefe JH Jr, Cordain L. Cardiovascular disease resulting from a diet and lifestyle at odds with our Paleolithic genome: how to become a 21st-century hunter-gatherer. **Mayo Clin Proc.** 2004; 79(1): 101-8. Review.

Rogerson D. Vegan diets: practical advice for athletes and exercisers. **J Int Soc Sports Nutr.** 2017; 14: 36.

Ruiz-Núñez B, Pruimboom L, Dijck-Brouwer DAJ, et al. Lifestyle and nutritional imbalances associated with Western diseases: causes and consequences of chronic systemic low- grade inflammation in an evolutionary context. **J Nutr Biochem.** 2013; 24(7):1183-1201.

Shai I, Schwarzfuchs D, Henkin Y, et al. Weight loss with a low-carbohydrate, Mediterranean, or low-fat diet. **N Engl J Med.** 2008; 359(3): 229-41.

Stanley S. **Children of the Ice Age** 1998; pp. 188-248. WH Freeman and Company.

Stryer L. **Biochemistry. (4th edition)** 1995; pp. 775-778. WH Freeman and Company.

Valencia ME, Bennett PH, Ravussin E, et al. The Pima Indians in Sonora, Mexico. **Nutr Rev.** 1999; 57: S55-S58.

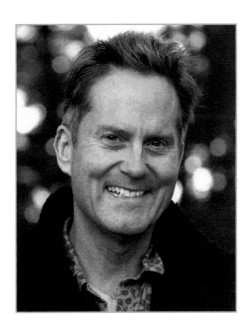

Rob Verkerk
BSc MSc DIC PhD FACN

As long as I can remember, I've been passionate about food and nature – and I've never seen the logic in keeping them separate. Hence my decision to study ecology at first degree level before continuing my academic journey with masters and doctorate degrees (Imperial College London), followed by a 7-year stint as a postdoc in agricultural sustainability.

As time went on, I increasingly felt the disconnect between agricultural and medical scientists. It never made sense to me that Western medics weren't more interested in using food as medicine, especially given the copious evidence to support its use. And why is medicine preoccupied with dealing with sickness, rather than with creating or regenerating health? Perhaps because I grew up in diverse African and Eastern cultures, I was more open from a younger age to the role of food on health than my academic colleagues? It was as if we spoke different languages.

Sustainable agriculture was all about working with nature, and applying learnings from stable, complex ecosystems like rainforests and coral reefs, to real-world farming systems. Ecological medicine existed but was in its infancy, being little more than a flea on the medical orthodoxy's back, scarcely being noticed. The year was 2002, and that's when I threw in the academic towel and decided to devote my energies into setting up the non-profit, the Alliance for Natural Health (ANH) International, as a vehicle for positive change, working to co-create health with nature.

Along my journey, like so many of us bearing the torch of 'food as medicine', I've been both harmed and healed by food. It wasn't until I quite radically changed my eating patterns, identifying then avoiding the foods to which I was intolerant, changing the way I prepared my foods, looked at foods as a source of information not energy, and became keto-adapted, that my health, resilience and vitality all came together. That was in my fifth decade of life, just as some of my peers were starting to wind down. Despite now being in my sixth decade, I feel a new dawn lies ahead of us. One in which we become inexorably engaged and respectful of natural systems, rather than chasing shiny new technologies that over-promise and under-deliver.

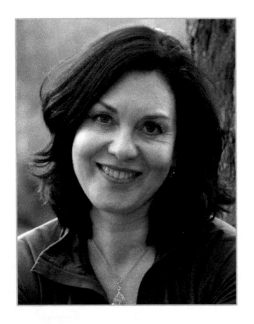

Meleni Aldridge

BSc NutrMed Dip cPNI Cert LTFHE

I spent the first 20 years of my life sick. A trauma in early life treated with years of drugs set me ricocheting between bouts of tonsilitis and gastro-enteritis. The latter was no surprise after the multiple courses of antibiotics year after year to treat the tonsilitis. By the time I reached 16, my resilience hanging by a thread, it was a short and swift descent into an autoimmune disease, but not without contracting glandular fever, quinsy, scarlet fever and dysentery on the way. A textbook journey to Grave's Disease. Yet not once was food ever even considered, either as a possible cause or for healing.

Having my entire thyroid removed at the age of 20, with the extent of unresolved metabolic dysregulation and inflammation I was experiencing, did not make me well. Quite the opposite. But it was the trigger for me to take back responsibility for my own health and it set me on a profound healing journey which has been extraordinary, enlightening, consciousness expanding and deeply heartfelt, for which I am now truly grateful.

Along the way I've practised many diverse healing modalities encompassing energy medicine and healing through to bodywork and nutrition, including receiving a BSc in Nutritional Medicine and a post-graduate diploma in Clinical Psychoneuroimmunology. My life's mission meshes so seamlessly with Rob Verkerk's and ANH that it was only a matter of time before our worlds collided back in 2002. I joined ANH full time in 2005.

Food and feeding are evocative and emotive because they are so integral to our survival as a species. But food is also one of the most powerful medicines I have encountered on my healing journey. Combining food and lifestyle interventions with finding your mission and purpose in life creates an effective prescription for much of what ails us. I hope the information in these pages helps you to also successfully push your metabolic reset button. The remainder we'll leave for another book.

©2022 ALLIANCE FOR NATURAL HEALTH INTERNATIONAL

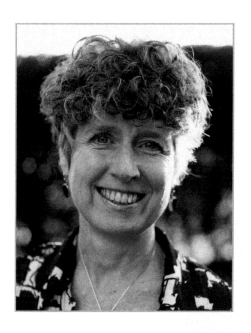

Melissa Smith
Dip ION

My passion for nutrition and cooking began as soon as I could stir a cake batter with my Nan. I learnt to cook from scratch at an early age and could feed a family of 6 by my teenage years. I continued to explore food and cook from scratch as I moved away from home but was soon seduced by the siren call of the supermarkets.

Fast forward 10 years and my health was on the floor. I discovered gluten and dairy free long before it went 'mainstream'. This sparked my love of recipe development and experimentation as I had to find other ways of feeding myself without the plethora of ingredients now available.

I continued my food and health journey by training as a nutritional therapist over 6 years ago, which led me to the door of ANH — the opening of a whole new world. The rest, as they say, is history!

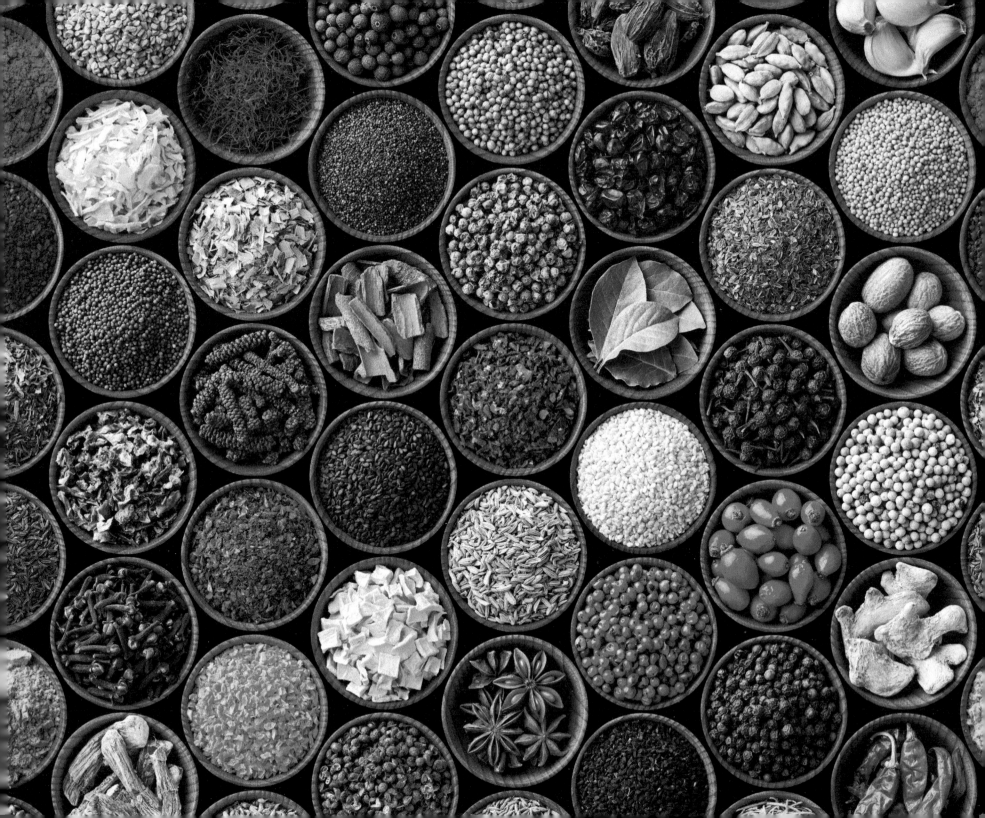